BLACK WOMEN'S HEALTH

Black Women's Health

Paths to Wellness for Mothers and Daughters

Michele Tracy Berger

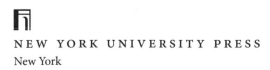

NEW YORK UNIVERSITY PRESS
New York

NEW YORK UNIVERSITY PRESS
New York
www.nyupress.org

References to Internet websites (URLs) were accurate at the time of writing. Neither the author nor New York University Press is responsible for URLs that may have expired or changed since the manuscript was prepared.

Library of Congress Cataloging-in-Publication Data
Names: Berger, Michele Tracy, 1968–   author.
Title: Black women's health : paths to wellness for mothers and daughters / Michele Tracy Berger.
Description: New York : NYU Press, 2021. | Includes bibliographical references and index.
Identifiers: LCCN 2020028152 (print) | LCCN 2020028153 (ebook) | ISBN 9781479828524 (cloth) | ISBN 9781479892952 (paperback) | ISBN 9781479876587 (ebook) | ISBN 9781479845422 (ebook other)
Subjects: LCSH: African American women—Health and hygiene.
Classification: LCC RA778 .B5234 2021 (print) | LCC RA778 (ebook) | DDC 613/.04244—dc23
LC record available at https://lccn.loc.gov/2020028152
LC ebook record available at https://lccn.loc.gov/2020028153

New York University Press books are printed on acid-free paper, and their binding materials are chosen for strength and durability. We strive to use environmentally responsible suppliers and materials to the greatest extent possible in publishing our books.

Manufactured in the United States of America

10 9 8 7 6 5 4 3 2 1

Also available as an ebook

CONTENTS

Introduction

I think one of the things that's been a problem for me is lack of support, like I have all these skinny friends who don't exercise, and it's fine for them, they feel like they don't need to exercise, which bums me out, but they're like why are you doing x, y, z? And you know I'm walking there [to the gym] . . . sometimes I'm the only woman of color there, so gosh, thanks, great. So that's sort of daunting sometimes in the gym, you know, and everybody's so happy to be there and I'm not really happy. . . . I think I lack the support . . . and people say you should exercise, but that's not really supportive. I mean it sounds supportive from afar, but it's really not supportive, sometimes it's like preachy. You should exercise. I know! Look at me, I know!
—Focus Group–Mothers

When I think of what makes a woman healthy, I think of choices—the choice to be positive, to be in control, the knowledge to sustain your body or at least even the knowledge to know what you should do . . . and some feeling of living in an environment that is safe and comfortable, and free of danger. Because I think there's health and then there's existing.
—Focus Group–Mothers

She [my mother] told me that I eat too much and I went to the doctor and [found out that I] . . . gained too much weight. So me and my mom had a conversation about eating healthy, but it didn't work.
—Focus Group–Daughters

I think health means that I feel happy about myself and I'm satisfied with myself . . . I don't really think that it's about how skinny I am or that kind of stuff. 'Cause I may be skinny . . . but I just may not be happy.
—Focus Group–Daughters

For the past decade, I have witnessed and recorded conversations about health and well-being by African American mothers and their daughters. Conversations between mothers were often animated, opinionated, engaging, and thought-provoking. The same was true in observing conversations between the daughters. The quotes above express central tensions and complexities of lived experiences that are often left out of the more common statistical presentations of health for African American women and girls.

Understanding how African American mothers and daughters discuss their health and what emerges from those discussions provides a window into the dynamic interplay between individual decisions and the structural forces that often assume an invisible role in shaping individual choices and preferences. Mothers in my study were asked the question: What is health? In each answer above, we get a glimpse into the individual experience and the possible structural forces that may exist in their lives that perhaps affect their ability to maintain their health (i.e., awareness of being a minority at a local gym, the importance of safety in relation to perceived neighborhood violence).

The last two quotes are from daughters in my study. They responded to the question: What conversations have you had with your mother about health? Analyzing the first response encourages us to be curious about what kind of cultural messages regarding weight and/or ideal body type the daughter may have been exposed to and how that mimics hearing a similar message about weight from her mother. And, we may also be curious about what it means to not get it *right* when it comes to health. What does healthy eating mean in this context? These are questions that deserve more attention. In the second response from a different focus group, we see that the speaker defines health as something positive and robust. And in thinking about this quote, our curiosity might be drawn to the word "skinny" and the ways that descriptor tells us something about girlhood and cultural norms. Our curiosity might allow us to consider the pointed messages that Black girls encounter regarding weight, how they may be susceptible to certain kinds of messages and may resist them in other instances. As I will discuss below, Black women's voices are infrequently theoretically centered in health literatures about how they experience and co-create their health, and it is even rarer for Black girls to be considered reliable knowers.

* * *

Medical and popular discourses shape much of what is known about Black women's and girls' health status. While African American women and girls show up repeatedly in broad national rankings and risk categories, researchers know little about the varied ways that African American mothers and daughters experience health as individuals or within family units. Moreover, we know even less about the quality and nature of health discussions that take place between African American mothers and daughters or how such discussions can, over time, affect health behaviors and outcomes.

This book evolved out of my experiences leading a team of researchers to explore mother-daughter communication, social support, and HIV risk. I began this work when North Carolina had the distinction of having the highest rate of HIV among southern states. One of the beautiful occurrences in research is when a project shifts in unexpected ways that demand new frameworks, skills, and abilities from the researcher. As the project moved on and deepened, it became less about HIV and more broadly about Black women's health and mother and daughter communication about health. It became examining the ways in which Black women and girls speak about and conceptualize health and well-being.

Black Women's Health explores the meaning and practice of health in the lives of African American women and their adolescent daughters. This work is developed through micro-theory that emerges from resonant themes from focus groups. Focus groups provide an organized way for researchers to convene everyday people and engage them in conversations of substance. Themes that I explore from the rich narratives include similarities and differences in external and internal barriers to health for mothers and their daughters, intergenerational legacies of caring, and the use of outdated gendered scripts by mothers in communicating about sexual health.

As I discuss below, this is timely work as both the study of Black women's and girls' health is being radically rethought by many scholars, and the public discussion and activism regarding Black women's and girls' well-being has become more visible in the last five years. What connects both developments is a call that Black women's and girls' complex lived experiences are integrated into research, policymaking, and activist agendas.[1]

This new direction in research especially constitutes an insurgent intervention because, as a group, African American women's health has never occupied a privileged place in America's health-care frameworks. As African-descended people, Black women's and girls' health has been shaped by and intertwined with the institution of slavery, Reconstruction, and post–World War II events that have positioned them as chronically and systemically situated low-wage workers and of lower social status than members of dominant communities. As many have documented, health care in the United States was not set up to support the flourishing of Black women and girls, and it continues to perpetuate staggering incompetence in both access and care resulting from the nexus of -isms, including but not limited to racism, sexism, classism, ableism, and heterosexism.[2]

Framing Questions and Goals of the Book

Black Women's Health explores the real-life meanings and everyday practices of health (i.e., mental, physical, emotional, and sexual) for the African American mothers and daughters whose narratives comprise the research.

The book draws from extensive fieldwork conducted with African American mothers and their adolescent daughters ages 12–18 in North Carolina pertaining to their discussions about health, sexuality, intimacy, and transitions to "womanhood" in a variety of contexts. My mixed-methods approach yields rich data that include interviews, participant observation, and focus groups. Focus groups help contribute to micro-theory.[3] In this case, micro-theory draws on multiple concepts to reveal patterns of intergenerational health practices and communication. The conversations presented in this volume take us beyond the statistics that simply collapse this group's experience into figures alone. By portraying the complexities of mothers' and daughters' daily negotiations of health realities, *Black Women's Health* presents an original collection of narratives that offer new dimensions of understanding how health is conceptualized, discussed, and practiced within this particular group.

This methodological framework draws from a Black feminist and intersectional theoretical orientation to situate Black women's and girls' health. *Black Women's Health* is thus the first scholarly book to treat the health status of African American mothers and daughters as integrally linked. Through a focus on women's and girls' narratives of health, and how they communicate with each other about the politics and practices of health, *Black Women's Health* probes the various ways in which African American mothers discuss these vital issues with their daughters, and how their daughters co-construct, interpret, and resist maternal and cultural narratives of health, sexuality, and racial identity. These direct accounts highlight how African American women and girls navigate their health and intimate relationships, as well as the various health inequalities rooted in the racism, sexism, and class marginality they experience.

Black Women's Health empirically extends existing scholarship by examining the range of communicative strategies that structure mother and daughter experiences of health and sexuality. *Black Women's Health* intervenes with a theoretical framework of intersectionality and Black feminist theory that seeks to situate a specific group of African American mothers' and daughters' health experiences in a southern milieu. A particular focus of the book is how African American mothers grapple with their personal health and sexual health histories and their daughters' health. In addition, the work is grounded in the standpoints of African American mothers and daughters and explores broad themes of intimacy, love, and relationships.

The framing questions of the book include: What can we learn by examining the health narratives of African American mothers and daughters? How do these health narratives present the multiple layers of African American mothers' and daughters' experiences of health, sexuality, intimacy, relationships, and risk for HIV/AIDS? And how does the sociological concept of "linked lives" as applied to health illuminate African American mother and daughter health experiences? [4]

Black Women's Health argues for understanding the importance of intergenerational dialogue between mothers and their adolescent daughters about health. Health is broadly defined and emerges from participants' definitions. It tackles both groups' concerns about their health and the health inequalities that are embedded in their daily lives. It also reveals the contemporary and ongoing struggles African American girls encounter on the path to developing healthy lives and intimate relationships. These kinds of conversations about health and sexuality between mothers and daughters have pointed implications for how daughters understand and respond to health risks, particularly for HIV and other STDs, and chronic health issues including obesity and diabetes.

Through a focus on communication, the book reveals the processes by which some African American mothers understand and shape the health trajectories for their daughters. This book demonstrates the multiple and conflicting messages about health that African American girls navigate at the critical point of adolescence. It also pays particular attention to the barriers to health that both mothers and daughters face. It highlights the ways some African American mothers use gendered scripts to engage daughters' sexual health, and how these scripts impact their daughters' understanding of their own health and health practices. This research reveals that some African American mothers may struggle with providing accurate and helpful sexual health information to their daughters, despite their overall desire to do so. Additionally, many mothers have not had an opportunity to process their own possible regret or challenges about their own sexual history, which may contribute to sending contradictory messages to their daughters about sexual intimacy.

Why Mothers and Daughters

The dynamic nature of intergenerational learning about health by focusing on the mother-daughter relationship is one of the original contributions of this work. I use the sociological concept of "linked lives" as an organizing frame for exploring mother and daughter relationships.[5] It is widely accepted that parent and child form a strong bond through social interaction, and that bond influences both parties throughout life.[6] Mother-daughter relationships support growth and development as well as growth and change. The dyad of African American mothers and daughters is a central focus for several reasons. Like other girls, African American girls construct their female identity in relationship to their mothers.[7] Similarly, African American mothers play a pivotal role in socializing their daughters into the complexities of young womanhood and identity development. Black mothering takes place within the sphere of inequality and that the socialization of daughters includes helping them navigate multiple and intersecting forms of oppression like race, class, and gender.[8]

For one, the health status for African American women and girls is marked by inequality in the areas of access, treatment, and resources; a focus on both through the dyad of mother-daughter relationships could yield important insights. There are other important demographic reasons why looking at mothers and daughters constitutes a useful focus. Demographically, Black mothers are more likely than other racial and ethnic minorities to head single-family households and also are more likely to head those families in the South.[9] Although there are other family configurations in the African American community, this is a central one. There are also widely documented health risks associated with single parenting.[10]

If we look only at the national health data for African American women and girls, we miss much of the context that can help us understand the unique barriers they face in the pursuit of health. We may also miss or devalue how resiliency, advocacy, and social support may play a positive role in African American women's and girls' health experiences. Using a more intimate approach can help researchers make visible the daunting role that structural inequalities play in shaping people's lives and provide insight into developing effective health interventions.

Black Women's Health offers such an approach. Its focus is on southern African American mothers and their adolescent daughters, and it examines the themes that emerge about health, information about and access to health and health care, and sexuality in a crucial period of girls' lives—early adolescence. It also pays particular attention to mothers' framing of intimacy, relationships, and ideas about HIV risk. The South continues to be a region that exhibits overall lower health status of its residents than the rest of the nation. African Americans in the South have higher rates of HIV/AIDS, diabetes, heart disease, and other diseases.[11] Moreover, the long-standing cultural taboos and silences about sexuality in the South continue to shape African American women's and girls' experiences.[12]

As one dimension of health, HIV/AIDS continues to be a vexing issue for policy makers and researchers alike. Rates of HIV infection among Black women in North Carolina reflect increasing rates of HIV infection in southern communities.[13] Poverty plays a significant role in shaping African American women's vulnerability to contract HIV.[14] Researchers know little, however, about how Black women, particularly in the South, and from different economic backgrounds, understand and assess their risk of contracting HIV.[15] We also know little about mother and daughter communication surrounding HIV. Thus, by delving into the daily experiences of African American mothers and daughters as they cope with, negotiate, and take action surrounding health, this book responds to many unanswered questions about mother-daughter communication regarding sexuality and HIV/AIDS awareness.

For example, we know that African American mothers employ sexual scripts in conversations with daughters, but we do not know enough about how these scripts affect their daughters' behaviors.[16] What do daughters find empowering or lacking in such scripts? How do these scripts prepare daughters for intimacy, and how do they raise awareness about various STDs? How can mother and daughter communication be strengthened to reduce HIV risk for both groups? My research provides the most comprehensive response to these questions to date, drawing from the population that faces the highest national health risk. From this data collected in North Carolina, *Black Women's Health* provides findings that are particularly salient for understanding the challenges in the region, while expanding the findings to address larger patterns that place African American women at such high health risks nationally.

As I discuss below, *Black Women's Health* fills an important void on health scholarship relating to African American girls and women. This is a timely discussion given the increasing focus on girlhood in women's and gender studies and calls to focus on African American girls in response to government initiatives such as *My Brother's Keeper* and the role of health in social movements, including Black Lives Matter and #SayHerName.[17]

No detailed book-length work privileges both components of the mother and daughter dyad and seeks to explore the bidirectional nature of learning and growth, specifically in the area of health.

Making Black Women's and Black Girls' Health Visible: Academic and Popular Frames

Black women's health does not belong to medicine, nursing or public health. We all have something to contribute to our survival. (Barlow and Dill 2018, 220)

The health realities of African American women and girls are not uplifting ones. By almost every criterion of fitness and mental and physical health, African American women and girls lag behind their white counterparts. African American women and girls experience both high rates of diabetes and low rates of physical exercise. African American women have the highest rates of being diagnosed as either overweight or obese of all groups in the United States: Approximately four out of five African American women are overweight or obese. African American girls are also disproportionately affected by obesity.[18] The statistics are startling, as one-quarter of African American girls ages 6–11 are obese (as compared with 14% of white girls) and 25% of African American female adolescents are obese (compared with 15% of white girls).[19] These figures reflect the challenging context in which African American girls mature into their own bodies and experience their health choices. They also provide a prism into the multidimensional factors that shape the context for decisions that African American mothers must make on a daily basis. From an intersectional perspective, these statistics reflect the larger landscape of racial and gender health disparities and structural inequalities.

Turning to African American women's and girls' sexual health, particularly concerning HIV/AIDS, the statistics are especially alarming. Despite a recent dip in 2010, the overall rates of HIV infection for African American women remain high. African American women account for 64% of new HIV infections among women, even though they constitute just 12% of the female population in the United States. African American girls, like other minority girls, also face high rates of HIV infection. The rates are especially high in the Deep South, which during 2008–2011 had the highest rates of HIV and AIDS diagnosis of any region in the United States. New trends suggest that one-third of all people living with HIV are in the South.[20] This disturbing new trend of rising rates of HIV in southern states also underscores long-standing issues of poverty and racial and gendered health disparities.

Much of what we know about Black women's health has come from academic inquiry, particularly through the fields of public health, social work, nursing, and to a lesser extent, sociology. Typically, much of the scholarship on Black women's and girls' health is quantitative, driven by biomedical frames. This scholarship historically tended to ignore context, intersectionality, regional variations, and the importance of intergenerational learning, especially in communities of color. Biomedical studies are unable—or less interested in—unpacking the contexts of domination and subordination in the structural arrangements through which health services are delivered and health is experienced. This work also does not often acknowledge the political contexts that influence how resources are distributed and the stereotypes, representational context, and discursive frames that may also affect how health is delivered.[21] Another criticism leveled at standard biomedical frames is that they remain focused primarily on individual behavioral change and are less focused on historical, community, and group experiences that many argue mediate health and reproduce health inequalities.[22] African American mothers' and daughters' health is not typically discussed or researched in connection to health disparities.

What's missing when we look only at the numbers? From a numerical perspective, there is a lot to know about the realities of African American women's and girls' health. However, from a critical theory, intersectional, and Black feminist approach, there is much to question. Self-identified Black feminist theorists, activists, and journalists have pioneered critical inquiry about African American women's health over the last three decades when most of academic inquiry ignored Black women's health.[23] Early work sought to identify the legacy of slavery, segregation, sexism, and classism as defining levers of Black women's experience of health and the legacy of health activism by Black women.[24]

When we look at Black women's and girls' health from only one dimension of analysis, we miss the rich legacy of theorizing that helps to bring about a robust analysis of how discrimination impacts Black women and girls. Black feminist approaches stem from the recognition that African American women experience the world through systemic and interrelated systems of oppression that include racism and sexism. The impact of these markers shapes power relations and creates unique experiences that differ in comparison with African American men or white women. As Patricia Hill Collins has identified, controlling images of African American women are shaped within power relations and have helped to produce the stereotypes of the Hottentot Venus, Jezebel, Mammy, Sapphire, and the more recent "baby mama."[25] There is a rich legacy of Black feminist theorizing that examines how representations of the Black female body, through various discourses, shape lived realities.[26] Black women's bodies have been historically devalued and governed by discourses of the grotesque, deviant, monstrous, disruptive, and masculine, or hypersexualized and subject to experiences of misogy-noir.[27] This legacy of representation stands in direct contrast to representations of white American women and African American men. These discursive frames of "normalcy" and "dominance" have long perpetuated Black women's "outsider" and "disabled" status.[28] Thus their "disruptive bodies" provide further justification for their devaluation and discrimination.[29] Scholars have used the frame of controlling images to examine media portrayals of African American women, perceptions about African American women and entitlement programs, the criminalization of African American women, as a feature of material culture of the antebellum South, and the social organization of motherhood.[30] Furthermore, Black feminist theorizing recognizes and seeks to document that African American women have a shared historical reality and thus, "a shared worldview of historical resistance to their own oppression and dehumanization."[31]

The dramatic picture of Black women's and girls' health calls for new tools, methodologies, and epistemologies beyond traditional approaches used in the applied and natural sciences (i.e., public health, nursing, etc.). Black feminist-driven approaches to health question the very tools and assumptions that have guided inquiry about health.[32] Turning to Black feminist epistemologies provides an opportunity to move beyond current tropes (i.e., "the strong Black woman" and hyper-resiliency) and familiar themes that are over-represented in the literature. Using Black feminist approaches, scholars have the opportunity to understand how trauma, resistance, and the legacies of racism and sexism affect Black women's and girls' health.

As Jameta Nicole Barlow and LeConté J. Dill note, the study of "Black women's health has too often been relegated to issues of sexual and reproductive health and chronic health conditions such as mental health, obesity, diabetes, hypertension and breast cancer. Yet our health encompasses so much more."[33] They do not argue that we ignore these overstudied areas and certain empirical findings, but that we advocate for a paradigm shift of what constitutes the study of health and who is qualified and encouraged to speak on it.[34] As I discuss in the next section, this movement in academic inquiry dovetails with the revitalization of Black women's health activism nationally and enriches the conversation. This new work is about grounding and context. Barlow and Dill's work follows scholars making ongoing recommendations for studies of Black women's health that employ methodological variety, represent the diversity within African American communities, and conduct research grounded in Black feminist theoretical insights.[35] Women's and gender studies analyses of Black women's health have more recently focused on reproductive politics and justice as well as on Black women's health and fitness regimes as part of identity politics and how African American girls navigate sexual scripts.[36]

My work methodologically and theoretically intervenes in the literature on racial and gender health disparities and moves this work into critical health studies and medical humanities, an interdisciplinary endeavor. This book contributes to conversations across various fields—most notably in sociology, public health, and women's and gender studies—about African American mothers' and daughters' health and sexuality. The majority of health literature on Black women treats the health status of African American girls and women as separate and rarely explores the connections between mother and daughter health.

This research also expands the sociological emphasis on Black families and the interdisciplinary interest in Black sexualities,[37] Black Girls' Studies,[38] and scholarly works on African American women's experiences of sexuality, love, and relationships.[39] It also engages intersectional questions about health.[40]

Discourses about Black women's and girls' health and well-being do not exist in a vacuum or solely within the domain of academics. I now turn to how African American women's and girls' health has been represented in popular culture during the past decade. I ask: What are the discursive and popular frames that shape African American women's and girls' health? There are three areas that are important to consider in framing aspects of Black women's and girls' health generally and mother and daughter health more specifically. I will briefly touch on Michelle Obama's "Let's Move" campaign (policy), the film *Precious*, the television shows *How to Get Away with Murder* and *Luke Cage* (media), and the activism of #SayHerName and Black Girl Magic interventions (social movements) and their influence in stimulating and shaping debates about race, gender, and health.

Health Warrior and Icon: Michelle Obama's Let's Move Campaign

Michelle Obama occupied a historic role as the first African American First Lady. The multiple roles that she claimed for herself—wife, mother, worker, and activist—were unique for a First Lady. One of her central and defining missions in that role was to "get America moving." As First Lady of the United States (FLOTUS), she specifically took aim at the ways in which Americans thought about their diet and sedentary lifestyles. Her 2010 Let's Move campaign sought to bring attention to childhood obesity and minimize the toxic environments in both the private and public spheres that contribute to childhood obesity. Her broader goal was to end childhood obesity in a generation.

Michelle Obama used her high-profile position to collaborate with an array of partners in government, medicine, science, business, education, and athletics that pledged to work together to get children "off their couches" and to consume fresher, healthier food. She consulted with a variety of health experts and policy makers and challenged grocers and city planners to add sidewalks to communities. She and President Obama used the creation of a community garden at the White House to inspire and underscore the importance of eating fresh fruits and vegetables as a pathway toward healthy living. Her vision stressed a multi-pronged approach that included individual changes for both parents and children, as well as changes at the structural level (e.g., nutritious school lunches and physical fitness programs, better availability of healthy foods in neighborhoods, along with neighborhood improvements including sidewalks). This multifaceted approach, while not without criticism, has often been minimized in critiques of her approach.[41]

Michelle Obama's communication and performance of health through her promotion of the Let's Move campaign initiated a new discursive space for mothers generally, and Black mothers specifically, linking health with motherhood, family, and even nation.[42] Her performance of fitness as a Black, middle-aged woman as desirable, and as achievable for some (especially for able-bodied and well-resourced women) was new. Despite justifiable criticism of aspects of the neoliberal framing of the Let's Move campaign, what has been missed is Michelle Obama's emphasis, in interviews and speeches, on pleasure, intimate connection, and joy in the pursuit of health for herself and her daughters. Her emphasis provides a distinct tension against the familiar and popular frame of individual and moral responsibility toward health. Moreover, Obama's comments about valuing well-being as defined by feeling good on the inside and not outward appearance intervenes in the standard tropes of addressing obesity and weight gain as a moral crisis.

Although there were many press stories about Michelle Obama's arms that objectified and sensationalized her body in a sexist way, Obama herself stressed her discipline in maintaining her exercise regimen which connotes accomplishment, yes, but also incrementalism, and more important, *prioritizing* pleasure and health over physical looks. She eschewed diets. She invoked pleasure and discussed what having a healthy body meant to her. Although she professed going to the gym often (and early), she also stressed the importance of pursuing fun as part of fitness, and even being silly, often remarking that "you don't have to be a great athlete to get out there."[43] She emphasized the pleasure she derived with her daughters as a core motivation, both for her own fitness and as an example for her daughters.[44]

It is still too early to assess the long-term results or impact of the Let's Move campaign, though some have argued that little substantive change was made in the policy realm to curb the decades-long lobbying efforts of certain corporate interests that oversee various food products and commodities that have been the beneficiaries of generous tax advantages and economic supports.[45]

Often the discursive space of health and wellness has been the terrain for white cisgender women, usually young and able-bodied. There are few spaces where African American women are positioned as experts and authorities on health, but Michelle Obama's influence in the public sphere contested those multiple dominant frames.[46] This was the first time that an African American woman had a public position that so thoroughly connected to and embodied a stance on health.[47] During 1993–1994, Jocelyn Elders, the Surgeon General during the first Clinton administration, was a public voice for health. However, she was widely criticized (and demonized) during her short tenure for her open discussions of safe sex and encouragement of masturbation. Because Michelle Obama occupied multiple roles in the American imagination, she was well-suited to a discussion on health. Her open embracing of both the joys and complexity of motherhood validated mothers, specifically African American mothers. As scholars have noted, African American motherhood has historically been devalued, with Black mothers most often being portrayed as incompetent.[48] Her health campaign relied on her public role as a mother (often referred to as the "First Mother in Chief"). This was a new moment for the country.

She credited much of her initial interest in creating a healthy lifestyle to her goal of "cooking a good meal for my kids."[49] She stressed how challenged working parents are, especially mothers, in facing the daily dilemma of meal preparation and cooking. Her interest in community gardens, fresh foods, and creating healthy meals was relatable to every working woman and especially mothers. President Obama is not absent in her discussions of cooking and the maintenance of family health, but Michelle Obama's role as a mother is centralized, which reinforces a gendered division of labor in the house and also in the domain of health.[50] Despite this more traditional positioning of motherhood, her story resonated so deeply because it struck many as true to many women's experiences.

In the past two decades, clinicians and public health scholars have warned the public about the obesity epidemic in the United States and globally.[51] Others have been critical about the framing of obesity, the resulting representation of who is obese, and the preponderance of neoliberal approaches that focus on individual versus structural solutions.[52] There were many ways

Michelle Obama's discussion of obesity left unaddressed the larger structural issues that also contribute to obesity, such as environmental pollution. However, Obama's statements also push back against framing obesity solely as a moral panic and crisis. Moreover, her comments shift the hyperfocus on weight and stigma that can become instilled in young people in particular, and instead stress emotional development and self-confidence.[53] Drawing on her experience raising her daughters, she presents a narrative less interested in policing the body. During interviews she repeatedly stated, "I never talked to them [her children] about weight in the household, we just started making changes . . . I just surrounded them with foods that were healthy and they could eat whatever they wanted . . . and just try to make activities fun."[54] In one interview, FLOTUS advised parents (and others) interested in modeling healthy behaviors for their kids to not "make this an issue about looks" but instead "talk to kids about how they feel inside." She argued that by doing so, people can look beyond "the physical manifestations of the challenge, but we're really tapping into what's going on inside the head of that child."[55] While naming an important and factual health issue—that one in two Black and Latino kids are obese and they will be disproportionately affected by diabetes— she periodically rejected the pervasive language of moral crisis and stigma. On this issue, she asserted, "we don't need someone to label it to know that we can fix it, we can change it."[56]

Although Michelle Obama's Let's Move campaign did not focus on African American women's and girls' health specifically, I argue her rhetoric of exercise as fun, as a way to connect to loved ones, and as pleasurable created a discursive space that resonated with many African American women and girls. Her alignment with Blackness and femaleness through mothering and defining her own body both encouraged and inspired many. Obama's health advocacy countered other negative public health messages that often framed Black women and girls as unfit and failed subjects. Given Obama's orientation to Blackness and femaleness, it is also therefore not surprising that while still promoting health during President Obama's second term, FLOTUS turned her attention to the issue of female empowerment and aligned herself with the extraordinary talent of pop superstar Beyoncé and many other Black women artists and cultural workers, making her message resonate globally.

Despite other limitations to Michelle Obama's approach, her representation of mothering and health echoes the women in this study (and the general public) who struggle to balance healthy family and healthy eating. The mother respondents saw themselves in that primary role, with diet, exercise, and weight manifesting as central issues in their discussions of that role.

Black Women's and Girls' Health in Film and TV

Film and television representations of Black women's and girls' health, especially in the context of mother (and mother-like figures) and daughter relationships, have had some important and key moments. The translation of the critically acclaimed novel *Push* by the writer Sapphire into the surprising, commercially successful film *Precious* marked a new cinematic moment for representing a wide variety of health issues in the African American community. Director Lee Daniels tackles subject matter that is not typical Hollywood fare. Daniels was the first African American male director to win an Oscar for a feature-length film award. The lead actress, Gabourey Sidibe, was nominated for an Oscar for Best Actress, and star Monique, who portrayed Precious's mother, won the Oscar for Best Supporting Actress. The film examines the legacy of intergenerational sexual trauma, violence of many varieties, and poverty. It follows Precious, the lead character, a dark-skinned, heavy-set young woman with almost no material resources, through a painful and difficult journey of self-discovery. The film raises many issues that are connected to health, including physical abuse, sexual violence, and obesity.

Much of the popular response in the African American community was divided, with some voicing their concerns that it reinforced stereotypes about Black parenting and demonized marginalized urban communities.[57] Others thought that it raised issues about color prejudice and structural inequalities in a particularly powerful, compelling, and aesthetically pleasing way.[58] I agree with Mia Mask's assertion that the film and its reception by both viewers and critics warrant a deeper reading beyond ideas of offensive or negative and positive representation.[59] The film provides opportunities for critical engagement with multiple facets of Black women's and girls' health. Precious's struggle with eating, sexual abuse, and being HIV-positive is particularly salient.

In the film, Precious faces the consequences of being sexually abused by both of her parents and contracting HIV from her father. Although the film, unlike the novel, tends to focus on the individual experiences of the character that are disconnected from structural conditions, it creates a place for the viewer to question the role of fast-food chain McDonald's and the ways in which healthy foods are unavailable to Precious and her community. The victimization of Precious and her response to stress by overeating and binging provide a corrective to the more popular notion that eating challenges are solely the domain of white and upper-middle-class women. The film also shifts the terrain away from the dominant discussions of bulimia and anorexia nervosa as the default way of understanding women's relationship with food and disordered eating and instead turns to "eating problems," as first identified by sociologist Becky Thompson in her work with a diverse group of women.[60] The eating problems that Thompson identifies through qualitative research are located within structures of oppression that the women face, including homophobia, classism, and racism. Investigating eating problems as an outcome of intersectional and complex factors gives space for fewer individualized diagnoses and greater community concern. As psychologist Susan Albers argues, "Precious's excessive weight and eating plays a central role in the movie. Aspects of the story help illuminate many of the reasons emotional, physical, and particularly sexual abuse, are risk factors for eating disorders."[61] In presenting Precious's struggle, the film challenges the more familiar narrative of control and morality, which are often central to the stigmatization of obesity, and instead shifts inquiry to the effects of intergenerational trauma.

Precious tackles familial sexual abuse and its connection to HIV. Precious is repeatedly raped by her father and sexually abused by her mother, yet she is blamed by her mother for her own victimization. The mother is as much a victim of long-sustained trauma as her daughter is, a portrayal that audiences do not often see. It raises complex issues of sacrifice and surrender. Like her father, Precious contracts HIV. HIV is still a major threat for African American communities, and this representation reignited discussion about the role of incest and sexual violence as a pathway for HIV, especially in lower-resourced African American communities. According to a 2016 study undertaken by Black Women's Blueprint, close to 70% of their participants had experienced sexual abuse before reaching the age of 18. Sexual violence in the home can be a pathway to HIV transmission. So, Precious represents a hyper-real cautionary tale about the intertwined legacies of sexual violence, HIV, and poverty.

In the last few years, we find similar tropes across television and film that include frank discussions about incest and sexual violence involving mothers and mother figures that are worth contemplating. Mother and daughter dynamics are at play on the popular TV series, *How to Get Away with Murder*, starring Viola Davis as Annalise Keating, the talented lawyer who is also an alcoholic and suffers from angry outbursts and possibly Post-Traumatic Stress Disorder. In the second season, it is revealed that Annalise was repeatedly molested by her uncle when she was a child. Her father was often absent because he was out of town and was an alcoholic. Cicely Tyson plays her mother and reveals that she knew that Annalise was being abused, although she did not acknowledge it at the time. As the season unfolds, it is made clear that her mother remedied the situation by setting the house on fire while the uncle was inside, killing him. Annalise is shocked and surprised by this revelation. This becomes part of the larger story and continues to unfold with a hostile confrontation with her father. What is interesting about this revelation is that the mother is unable to understand why Annalise might still be angry and upset, as if that one major act would absolve all of her daughter's complex emotions.

In the third season, Annalise had a major reversal of fortune when she was placed in jail on suspicion of murder. She confronts her father while in jail by revealing that his brother molested her. She suggests that she understands the connection between past and current trauma by saying, "You think *that* has nothing to do with me being here?" He deflects and states, "We are all in pain." By leveling her comment, it puts the viewer in the role of sympathizing with the father and with the status quo. It minimizes the impact of sexual trauma and reduces it to another kind of pain without recognizing and encouraging a more empathetic view. A more empathetic view does not excuse Annalise from her many misguided (and often criminal) actions but would allow for a nuanced consideration of the costs of living with this secret and the shame it engenders. Such consideration would also highlight how her history of sexual abuse explains the context of her other intimate relationships, like her marriage to a husband who cheated on her and her inability to emotionally connect with lovers. The show does present these as connected, but I would argue it does not fully challenge the more status quo assumption that sexual assault can "just be gotten over with" without a long-term engagement. Early in the season, Annalise does not reveal her experience of sexual violence to anyone outside of her family sphere. At times she recognizes she is a survivor but is unable to consciously act on that knowledge and seek help. Season 3 depicts a reversal of these trends when her father acknowledges her trauma, and although Annalise begins to refer to what has happened to her, still she struggles with shame and self-loathing.

Others have written on the mental health of Annalise and the threads of the "Black Superwoman" stereotype that, despite ongoing trauma "suffered at the hands of her husband, family and even students, she continues to march on," advancing her career and helping others.[62] The character is portrayed as super tough, both by her own naming and the way others see her. Those around Annalise both vilify and exalt her for these traits, which feeds into the trope of the isolated strong Black woman. Nsenga Burton goes on to argue that for some viewers, watching this character can reinforce the very real-world idea "that seeking professional help, attempting radical self-care, or taking time to heal from trauma is of no benefit to Black women."[63] I would agree that in seasons one and two of the series, a struggle exists between representing the view that childhood sexual abuse can and does have a long-term impact on mental and physical health and the view that a survivor's revelation and disclosure within the family is sufficient.

Despite the show's inconsistent narrative, I would argue that the viewer comes to recognize that Annalise is increasingly unable to cope and, despite her outward bravado, the challenges of shame, low self-worth, and trauma related to sexual violence threaten to destroy her and cannot be justified as simply being about her personality. Indeed, her journey through season three is one of recovery and redemption. This trend continues in seasons four and five, and offers through backstory the deep challenges of shame, low self-worth, and trauma that define Annalise.

Although it is not uncommon for television shows to portray incest and childhood sexual abuse, it is striking that two very different and popular shows, both featuring Black actresses, have played with this theme in the last few years. In the Netflix production of *Luke Cage*, politician Mariah Dillard, played by Alfre Woodward, carries resentment toward her aunt who raised both her and her cousin Cornell "Cottonmouth" Stokes, played by Mahershala Ali. As the story evolves, there is notable tension and antagonism between her and Cottonmouth. They were raised in the same household by an aunt and uncle who were involved heavily in crime. Cottonmouth believes that she was favored, but what is revealed to the audience is that she was moved out of the house and sent to boarding school to avoid additional sexual violence by her uncle. Mariah harbors deep resentment because she felt removed from the family and abandoned, forced to adapt to a different community and culture in boarding school. Toward the end of the first season, in a heated encounter and argument between her and Cottonmouth, he says, "You enjoyed it." This is an odious comment, yet often a common experience that survivors must learn to cope with. She, in a moment of blind rage, strikes him and he loses his balance and is thrown through an office window, falling several stories from the balcony. Mariah, who has accidentally caused his fall, continues to rage as she comes downstairs, and in a spectacular and excessive amount of force, repeatedly strikes him and screams, "I didn't ask for it." Others have written about this moment as one that serves to allow the character (and audience) to recognize that she is a killer despite her well-groomed self-image.[64] I argue there is something more that resonates with the viewer that is specific to the nature of the offense. Telling the truth breaks something loose that is both ugly and cathartic for the character and the spectator. This strikes me as a powerful moment that replays the larger narrative of women, especially Black women as sexual survivors wanting and inviting their abuse and stands out as a powerful counternarrative.

In surveying this celluloid terrain, what is striking are the less common depictions of the struggles that many women in my focus groups face with their own health challenges, including managing diabetes, chronic heart conditions, the rigors of learning new recipes for a healthier diet, or the concerns they have about keeping their daughters at a healthy weight. We see fewer depictions of everyday health challenges that mark many African American women's and girls' experiences of health. We also see few depictions of the racial and gender health disparities that map onto Black women's experiences accessing medical care, which is also a theme among respondents. While it is notable that important health issues like HIV and sexual violence (and, increasingly, mental health issues)[65] are becoming more common in media, there are still several gaps in representation of the mundane and daily health issues faced by many.

Black Women's and Girls' Activism Intersecting with Health

In the year 2015, several Black women activist groups showed the power of Black women: #Blacklivesmatter #Sayhername, #SandraBland, #BreeNewsome are movements to claim Black women's rights as human rights.[66]

In the last five years, the political terrain has exploded with activism led by Black women and Black girls articulating the structural realities they face. Responding to the multifaceted threats on Black Life, including police brutality, sexual violence, and political viability, has brought issues of Black women's and girls' health into popular focus. There is a recognition that ongoing legacies of trauma and violence impact Black women's and girls' mental, physical, and spiritual well-being. The year 2015 was a watershed moment, as Evans notes above, and Black women's activism has continued. We can also include Tamara Burke and the founding of the #MeToo movement in this explosion.

Black Lives Matter brought to the forefront issues of police brutality and the failures of the criminal justice system, while challenging the narrative of a post-racial America. Within the context of organizing, Black women systematically challenged their own exclusion from being seen as worthy victims. Within the context of this discussion, a broader political space emerged that examines the ways in which Black girls' lives are devalued.

Activists and scholars have offered a chilling picture of the state of Black girls' well-being in the United States. Black girls tend to battle greater stressful life events than many of their counterparts. For instance, the Girl Scouts's 2013 State of the Girls report found that Black girls are more likely than any other members of racial or ethnic groups to: live in single-parent households, report being hit by a boyfriend, and be overweight or obese. Additionally, this group has a teen birth rate two times that of the national average and has a poverty rate that is double that of white girls. The 2019 report, "Girlhood Interrupted: The Erasure of Black Girls Childhood," presents evidence demonstrating that Black girls face the distinct challenges of being seen as more mature and less innocent by adults.[67] Black girls are less likely to be viewed as deserving to be treated (and protected) as children. Authors of the report argue that this level of "adultification"[68] puts Black girls at risk for various kinds of violence. A particularly egregious example of this kind of perception is the treatment in 2015 of Dajerria Becton, the fifteen-year-old Black girl who was slammed down to the ground at a pool party by Eric Casebolt, a police officer.

Black girls are also vulnerable in many institutions, including schools. Kimberlé Crenshaw, gender and racial equity pioneer, co-authored a report titled, "Black Girls Matter: Pushed Out, Overpoliced and Underprotected," that highlights the ways that schools reinforce sexism and racism and thus reduce Black girls' educational opportunities. This report, which received major press, highlights how schools curtail their "educational opportunities, and marginalize their needs, while pushing them into low-wage work, unemployment, and incarceration."[69]

These negative patterns and their impact definitely do not contribute to the flourishing of Black girls' well-being. Crenshaw critiques the focus on young Black boys and systemic oppression with policy remedies that are not intersectional and that overlook the needs of Black girls. Refocusing on Black girls and women through policy and community, as Crenshaw argues, helps us mobilize creativity and energy to find solutions that do not replicate traditional patriarchal norms.[70] In this vein, some scholars are building creative interventions based on a strength and resiliency model of Black women's and girls' experiences.[71] These interventions often have well-being and health at their center. African American female digital activism has been particularly powerful as it emphasizes well-being, self-care, and health as part of a political orientation.[72]

The rise of #BlackGirlMagic as a recent set of aesthetic and activist practices reveals the multiple and creative ways Black girls and women use poetry and other creative expressions to counter negative experiences and engage resistance. The social movement began in cyberspace but has since evolved to encompass organizing practices and spaces offline. Julia Jordan Zachery and Duchess Harris explore how #BlackGirlMagic is an articulation of the multiples ways in which "Black femmes, women and girls" make themselves visible and legible using creative methodologies, representations, and practices within the face of structural oppressions.[73]

These important developments continue to shape the discursive and political terrain about the meanings and practice of health for Black women and girls.

Methods

My investigation into how African American mothers and daughters discuss and experience issues of health draws on focus group interviews and field research conducted between 2004 and 2010. The community of respondents were 24 pairs, each composed of a self-identified African American mother and her identified daughter. I was deliberate about construing the identifiers "mother" and "daughter" as broadly as did my respondents, to accommodate nontraditional, less formal, and nonbiological mothering relationships.[74] The daughters that were recruited were between the ages of 12 and 18. The average age of the mothers was 35. The average age of the daughters was 14. There were five mother focus groups and five corresponding daughter focus groups, for a total of 48 participants. Each of the mother and daughter focus groups were conducted on different days. The appendix provides more demographic information about the study participants and additional methodological notes.

The focus groups took place in a variety of locations, including public libraries and community centers. When mothers and their daughters arrived at the study site, daughters were escorted to one room and their mothers were escorted to another room. They had separate semi-structured conversations organized around a set of questions defined primarily by several themes—health and wellness, adolescence, mother and daughter relationships, and experiences with health-care providers. I alternated at times between being a facilitator and moderator across mother and daughter groups. Taking on these roles gave me different vantage points throughout the research period. The focus groups usually lasted for two hours to two and half hours, sometimes longer.

As Richard Krueger notes, this process in focus groups is evolutionary for participants and as research unfolds, that influences how the researchers conceptualize their work.[75] As I began this research, my preference was to keep questions broad and allow them to "ripen" and develop over time. For example, I asked the mothers generally: What have they shared with their daughters about becoming a young woman? This question evolved to having the mothers tell us what they have shared with their daughters about the idea of intimacy and how they might envision their daughter's first date. Thus, although the majority of questions were asked of all groups, some were probed further in some instances and others not as much. I note this in the analysis.

Focus groups were transcribed and then coded by me. After identifying major and recurrent themes and patterns, I performed detailed coding of the data. This involved several readings of the transcripts from each focus group, paying attention to one particular dimension each time (e.g., exercise). Each time I read through transcripts and my notes, I became more and more intrigued with how mothers (in the mother groups) and daughters (in the daughter groups) talked about their definition of health as well as their reflections on conversations about the same topics in their families. I read the transcripts to cross-check themes, their interior layers, and emerging contradictions.

Drawing on grounded theory and informed by my knowledge of literature on the topic, I concentrated on exploring the themes that emerged inductively from the focus groups and field notes. I also worked to understand the perspectives of the participants being expressed and paid attention to the complex ways that mothers, in particular, influenced each other, changed their narratives, and revealed their hopes and dreams for themselves and their daughters.

Analysis

Focus groups have historically occupied a rather "stepchild"-like status within the spectrum of qualitative methods, often viewed as lacking the rigor and depth of one-on-one interviews. Focus group research is often viewed as a straightforward, economical, and less intensive research methodology. This perspective has been recently challenged by many, including feminist scholars who argue that focus groups analysis,[76] when it moves away from a strict positivist and market research frame, offers important ways to explore the collective and interactive nature of the production of subjectivity. Focus groups can also allow for debate, disagreement, and thoughtful group reflection that can undermine, challenge, or even subvert researchers' categories and assumptions about the group.[77] They also provide the potential for sharing power in the research process and establishing principles of feminist ethics.

In presenting focus group data methodologically, much of the interaction, contradiction, and interpersonal dynamics are left out or minimized in reporting and analyzing focus group data.[78] I am in interested in both the "how" and the "what" that comprise my focus groups. The "how" is the interactional processes that mothers and daughters created in their respective focus groups. The "what" is the content and meaning that developed out of the focus groups. In *Black Women's Health*, I use the richness of focus group material to tease out several layers of meaning. I draw on conversational and narrative analysis at the group level—a key strength of focus group data. The focus groups were different in ways that the participants engaged each other, the moderators they had, and the conclusions that they reached throughout the time together. I note areas of clarity, confusion, and disagreement among participants. Where relevant, for the mothers' groups, I draw on health status, profession, and marital status and other important markers of the conversation.

I pay less attention to individual statements and instead focus on thematic concerns and how ideas are developed through interaction in a group and then across groups. This means looking at how the groups of mothers and their daughters differ. I am then able to analyze all the mother groups in total, all the daughter groups in total, and also make comparisons *between matching* mother and daughter focus groups, thus adding another level of analytical richness. I also pay particular attention to the group interaction that occurred in the mothers' groups as it governs my broader interest in how conceptualizations of health are communicated between mothers and daughters.

Taking note of group-level dynamics and including that in one's analysis is unconventional in focus group research. Wendy Duggleby, however,[79] notes that "group interactions are a source of data that is underused and underreported in focus group research." Paying close attention to the context of group dynamics can offer analytical insights that would otherwise be missed. For example, I noticed that in almost all of the mother focus groups, the mothers engaged each other directly on sensitive issues of health and sexuality and shared experiences that promoted group rapport. They often talked over the moderator and offered each other resources and support, which surprised us. Later, my research team and I reflected on why so few public or private spaces exist for Black mothers from differing backgrounds to come together and share a diversity of experiences about difficult and contested issues (e.g., daughters' sexual experiences). This allowed me to question the structural factors that prevent African American women's forums from discussing issues of mothering, health, and sexuality in a safe, nonjudgmental setting. And, finally, it allowed me to ask: How can communities encourage innovative forums that support skill-building and support for Black mothers on difficult and complex issues? It is from this conceptual framework and its complementary methodological approach that the structural framework for this book emerges.

There are multiple approaches to analyzing focus groups and little agreement among them. Despite the lack of coherence about analysis of focus groups, there are three main recurring concerns that need to be addressed. They are conformism, length, and the iterative nature of the questions. I address them here.

Members of focus groups can arrive at consensus too quickly and reflect levels of conformism about a topic that may run counter to their observations and preferences. This was not the case for the participants in my focus groups, especially the mothers. African American women rarely have a time to meet and talk with others about their health needs and concerns about their daughters. All the focus groups were highly engaged and typically did not display signs of conformism about topics. There were a few instances in the daughter groups where consensus emerged quickly. The composition of the ages of the daughters' groups ranged, so it might have been the case that in certain instances, younger girls may not have spoken up as frequently or forcefully as their older counterparts. They also might have come to consensus from a lack of experience on the topic, lack of knowledge, or discomfort discussing certain subjects in the study setting. Overall, as I note in chapter 1, daughters were highly engaged and enthusiastic participants and thus there was no significant discernable pattern related to age. The guide that we used asked questions from multiple vantage points, thus minimizing the chance of a more homogenized outcome.

The second concern often raised about focus groups is the length of reporting. Focus group reporting produces voluminous data. A key issue becomes representation. If we err on the side of concision, then we can miss the very context of the conversation that supports the researcher's analytical argument.[80] It is more dangerous to summarize and compress so much of the data that the interaction, one of the vital aspects of this method, is flattened and lost. It is also possible to go so far in the other direction that the reader loses the centrality of an analytical point while wading through pages of conversation that wanders across many different topics. This approach can fatigue the reader. I have erred on the side of longer and more robust quotes throughout the book. My goal was to present the reader with enough of the context of the conversation to provide a road map for how components of the conversation were analyzed.[81] I also give clear signals about when and why I am focusing on the interactive nature of the discussion.

The third concern is what counts as enough in the reporting of themes comparing multiple focus groups. I rely on Jaime Harding's suggestion that themes were further explored and developed if they appeared across one-fourth of the groups.[82] In this case, I used the standard of three of the five groups (both for mothers and daughters). This seemed to be both common-sensical and a valid goal for making claims that work beyond the set context of groups. Working within these constraints, there are times I stray to follow the unique perspective of a group as an outlier among the others. The tension between exploring the value of what emerges in one group versus multiple groups is something that I wrestled with throughout the analysis.

Finally, a key piece of thinking through the "what" of the findings is the analytical approach undergirding the work. Black feminist scholarship and intersectional research attend to the social location of the researcher (e.g., race, class, and gender), look at relationships of power from multiple dimensions, and reveal systems of power that can be micro- or macro-focused.[83]

Intersectionality as an analytical tool also helps me to both highlight that African American mothers' and daughters' narratives about health have not featured prominently in research—thus providing a context to understand hidden or marginalized experiences—and bring attention to how unmarked categories of health, gender, and power are contributing to the lived experiences of African American women and girls. For example, the discourse on healthy exercise is often presented in a way that suggests equal access (to gyms and workout facilities, in schools, workplaces, or homes) is the preferred and most important approach coupled with individual responsibility. Bringing an intersectional approach that examines more critically how this formulation assumes a class advantage and ignores other possible barriers (i.e., the internal feelings from being a minority in a majority-dominated gym) puts into context some of the mothers' (and to some degree daughters') challenges in seeking to be "fit." Hae Yeon Choo and Myra Marx Ferree note the limitation of intersectional work that only seeks inclusion.[84] Instead, they encourage researchers to make visible how dominant unmarked categories shape individual and group experiences. This intersectional work calls attention to African American women's and girls' health narratives not just as a "special kind of difference" (than, for example, white women and girls), but to interrogate the structural (and discursive) social organizing principles that shape Black women's and girls' health practices.[85]

Organization of This Book

Chapter 1. Mother and Daughter Narratives about Health, Sexuality, and Young Womanhood

This chapter presents general patterns about the relationships between southern African American women and their adolescent daughters with a focus on health, well-being, sexuality, and HIV/AIDS as topics that emerge from the data. It also provides an overview of how daughters experience communication with mothers. I situate the health status of African American girls and women in North Carolina during the study period. I introduce a narrative typology of the focus groups. My typology of the mother and daughter focus groups is presented with specific characterizations to help readers distinguish among each group and how their "worldview" reflected particular themes. These central tenets form guiding strands throughout the book. For example, one group is labeled "Experts" because of the ways the group articulated the choices they made about how they discussed health-related issues with their daughters. It also refers to the way that they positioned themselves in the context of their expertise as health professionals. I highlight the themes that are connected to young womanhood for daughters, of respect, trust, and pressure.

Chapter 2. Mothers' Health Narratives

How mothers define health, their health experiences, and expectations for themselves and their daughters are front and center in this chapter. It also investigates the ways that mothers communicate expectations about their daughters' health. Four themes emerge in the mothers' narratives of health: (1) mothering practices of health, (2) implicit and explicit barriers to health, (3) how race and gender inform their experiences navigating health care, and (4) their perceptions of risk of daughters' health.

I examine several areas of narrative tension for mothers in how they discuss their health practices with their daughters and represent those practices to themselves. I capture the concept of legacies in mother and daughter communication and how mothers either borrow, incorporate, or reject communicative styles and patterns from their mothers. Mothers had a tendency to characterize themselves in opposition to their own mothers and grandmothers regarding health-care access, sexuality, and general openness of communication. These generational differences reveal how both their health and wellness are shaped by the ongoing legacies of the Jim Crow South and the shifting configurations of power, exclusion, segregation, and resistance.

Chapter 3. "I'm in Between": Daughters and Health Inheritances

The multiple ways that daughters define health and how they think about their own health needs is the focus of this chapter. Identifying the meaning of health elicited a broad range of answers from the daughter groups—everything from "hygiene" to "responsibility." Health-care access, perceptions of doctors' treatment of them, and their own struggles to stay healthy are explored. Their narratives reflect present-day challenges for many young teens, including the lack of consistent physical activity, access to cheap and unhealthy foods, and the financial struggles of working parents. Although many of the daughters have been exposed to a great deal of health information and health-care access, they often do not see or experience themselves as healthy. Their narratives also indicate areas of strength and resilience in girls' awareness of the media's role in circulating unrealistic body images.

Chapter 4. "I Want That First Kiss to Be Perfect": Mothers on Intimacy, Pleasure, and Sexuality

This chapter looks at how mothers grapple with communication about sexuality and intimacy. Mothers' fears and insecurities about how their daughters will negotiate relationships and sexuality distinctly emerge in these narratives. In discussing their concerns about their daughters, their own sexual stories and the challenges they experienced with their parents and peers (but most especially their mothers) are revealed. The chapter explores how mothers grappled with and confronted their own past sexual histories and challenges, or did not. The contexts of intimacy and desire are investigated as mothers frame loss and possibility in their hopes for their daughters' intimate lives. We also begin to see how single-parent status and being an early mother influence patterns of communication across groups.

Chapter 5. "Mom, Can We Talk about Sex?": Daughters and Sexuality

What are the things that daughters would most like to know about relationships, intimacy, and sexuality from their mothers and adult female figures? What is the social landscape regarding sexuality, and what mixed messages do daughters have to navigate? Who do they turn to when they have questions about sex and intimacy? This chapter explores all of these questions.

I demonstrate that there is a mismatch with mothers' perceptions of easy and open communication about sexual health and sexuality with their daughters and what daughters express. Although many mothers saw themselves as more open and receptive to talking about sexual health (and health in general) compared to their own mothers, daughters did not believe they could get accurate, nonjudgmental information from their mothers. Daughters expressed the desire for information and skill-building around communication. The potential health consequences for daughters given challenges in mother and daughter communication are explored.

I argue that responses to a scenario posed to daughters reveal the ways in which gendered behavior shapes and constrains their expectations about male and female relationships and illuminates the micro-dynamics of gender.

Chapter 6. Resolutions

The conclusion ties together the various strands of the book's argument and demonstrates that scholars, public policy officials, and African American communities all have important roles to play in changing the complex picture of African American women's and girls' health. I argue that, in order to make an impact on the health and well-being of African American women and girls, scholars must understand the contextually rich experiences of mothers and daughters. Patterns about mother and daughter communication and how they navigate intersecting forms of oppression provide important places to look for clues about health practices and can play a role in structuring interventions and improving medical provider interactions. When we ask different questions about the experience of health of African American mothers and their adolescent daughters with a more nuanced and qualitative approach, we see more of both the challenges and the possibilities. The resiliency of how Black girls work to maintain their health while navigating gender and racial stereotyping is more clearly captured by this approach. This research broadens our understanding of how African American girls interpret, cope with, and push back against both familial and cultural messages of health and well-being. Public policy debates across several dimensions, including health, sexual education, and HIV/AIDS, are discussed to provide a context for strategic planning and thinking. I also offer ideas about the role that communities can play in supporting African American mothers' caretaking and the need for broader public investment in African American girls.

1

Mother and Daughter Narratives about Health, Sexuality, and Young Womanhood

This book explores the health narratives that circulate between a core group of African American mothers and their daughters. The daughters are within a crucial age range, 12–18 years old. The transition from girlhood into young womanhood is one of change and transformation. The territory of the self dramatically changes during this time, both physically and emotionally. New marks and blemishes appear on one's skin, hormonal changes demand attention in defining the body, the ease of childhood delights fades and questions about what is emerging in this new skin and body come to the fore. How will it act? What will it want? One's moods begin to become unpredictable, and then on top of these personal changes come the social changes. A flood of questions often bubble up in young girls, including: What kinds of things am I good at? Whom do I like? What does attraction feel like? Should I go out with this person? What does it mean to date? What do I love about school? Who are my true friends? Should I worry about my weight?

The girls in the focus groups wrestled with identity, body image, health issues, and navigating peer and romantic relationships. They spoke openly about what it meant for them to be healthy. Mothers are also struggling with decisions that have serious ramifications, including: When should my daughter start dating? What should I tell her about my own past? What is the appropriate level of communication?

This chapter has two main goals. The first goal is to introduce readers to the mother and daughter focus groups. The second goal is to provide an overview of the general patterns of communication between these mothers and daughters. Who are these mothers and daughters at this turning point? How do they think about young womanhood? What are the ways that communication is perceived between them? I am specifically concentrating here on mothers' perceptions of their daughters' journey into womanhood, as those themes about health and sexuality shape much of the book.

I accomplish this through creating a narrative typology of mothers' and their corresponding daughters' "worldviews" based on their focus group sessions. Throughout the book I will be talking about how these focus groups (and the themes that arise from them) comprehensively draw analytically on these worldviews. This chapter provides the opportunity to experience each focus group as a unique collective. By naming and describing each one, I hope to anchor some key features about the groups' dynamics in the reader's mind. I have also provided a table that provides a quick visual reference point.

The mothers' worldview tells us something about their orientation to their health, their daughters' health, sexuality, and general well-being. The worldviews also differentiate their approach to viewing the challenges and opportunities facing them. It encapsulates a dominant narrative arc they embodied during the focus group conversation. The worldviews are based on narrative tension, repetition, and how the respondents engaged others. Using this worldview framework also captures the embodied nature of the underlying energy of the conversation and performative nature of group interaction. Thus, voice, emphasis, emotion, body language, and energy level all contribute to my understanding of meaning that was created in the group and they are the building blocks of my analysis.

The worldviews of the mothers drive much of the discussion throughout chapter 2 and chapter 4. The mothers' worldviews set the context for understanding how daughters translate their mothers' communication and health behaviors. So, for example, there are the Experts, the Transitioners, the Revealers, the Nostalgics, and the Strategists. The "experts" emphasize authority and assurance, the "transitioners" are about change and managing change, the "revealers" are focused on disclosure, the "nostalgics" concentrate on learning from personal history, and the "strategists" are all about finding techniques and best practices to manage daughters' transitions into womanhood. Analytically, the worldviews serve another purpose in that they also capture how the mothers understand (or don't understand) patterns in their lives (e.g., being "in transition"). The daughters in turn are discussed as the Romantics, the Equalizers, the Loners, the Moderates, and the Distrusters. These worldviews reveal their orientations to their health, perceptions of their mothers' health, and trust regarding issues of sexuality and communication with their mothers. Their worldviews are the foundation for discussion in chapter 3 and chapter 5.

As stated in the introduction, my analysis is less interested in tracking individual narratives and more interested in examining themes that emerge in each group and across groups. As much of my methodological focus is to illuminate group-level dynamics of focus groups and to reveal how this yields analytical insights, this typology foregrounds themes of mother and daughter health issues that will be developed in subsequent chapters. Any typology created confers a sense of neatness, linearity, and finality. The goal is to present patterns that emerge and mark a clear territory but does not close off other ways of viewing the material.

The benefit of having the groups organized around individual focus groups that convened (as opposed to organizing solely around singular analytical themes that draw on individual speakers) is that I am able to explore rich interaction and group dynamics. This reveals how *mothers talk among themselves* and how *daughters talk among themselves* about key issues. I'm also able to analytically link up corresponding mother and daughter groups, for example, the Experts (mothers) and the Equalizers (daughters), and probe the way events, concepts, and histories are narrated, exposing interesting frictions that yield important dimensions of mother and daughter communication. Insights into intragroup and intergroup dynamics are a major strength of this approach.

Second, this chapter's goal is to present general patterns of communication between mothers and daughters and the main theoretical themes about health, well-being, sexuality, and HIV/AIDS that emerge from the data. This chapter sets the tone for the book by providing an overview of how daughters experience communication with mothers, their experiences with health, and young womanhood. Although the themes are presented across three different areas, there is much overlap in narratives about health that also touch on sexuality, sexual identity, ideas about sexuality, and gender identity. Each of these themes is discussed further in depth in subsequent chapters.

Before meeting the mothers and daughters, we will consider the local health conditions in their place of residence.

African American Women's and Girls' Health in North Carolina

Looking more closely at the health indicators during the last decade, a period that covers the duration of the study, we see challenges in the status of African American women's and girls' health, as discussed both generally and more specifically in North Carolina. North Carolina is embedded in a region of the southern United States that has been a hotbed of poor health, often consistently ranked lower in comparison with other regions. This includes higher rates of cancer, diabetes, and heart disease.[1]

The Center for Women's Health Research, part of the University of North Carolina at Chapel Hill's School of Medicine, provides a report card on the state of women's health in North Carolina, examining several key areas including infant mortality, barriers to health, chronic disease, and reproductive health. Beginning before the study period in 2007 and spanning two years past the study period in 2012, we see consistent declines in health for African American women and girls. The percentage of African American women who were obese and who had diabetes, high cholesterol, heart disease, high blood pressure, and had suffered a stroke all increased by two to five percentage points.[2] Barriers to health increased from 2007 through 2012, including a two-percentage-point increase among Black women without health insurance and Black women who were unemployed. Turning to infectious diseases like HIV, we find that North Carolina also had among the highest overall rates of HIV in the South and in the country during the time of the study period.[3] Although there were slight decreases for other groups (especially Native American women) during this period, HIV rates remained steady for Black women. During this time, however, Black women's rates of HIV remained 14 times higher compared to white women.

These indicators remind us that the health of Black women in North Carolina, like the rest of the country, has been and continues to be a cause for concern and investigation. The structural inequalities including class, race, and gender that shape North Carolina Black women's realities form a pattern and template for African American women and girls across the United States.

Mothers

The Experts

Experts expressed confidence as they gave their answers and the way that they discussed their communication with their daughters. Their narratives stressed expertise (often specialized knowledge that stemmed from professional identity), certainty, and assuredness. As compared to the other mother focus groups, their answers were often straightforward and conveyed less doubt, reservation, and emotional turmoil. The Experts simply did not wrestle with questions about their own and their daughters' sexuality and health in the way that characterizes other groups.

Given that the group includes a medical doctor and two health educators, we might expect that these mothers would have salient and sophisticated ideas about health care and health delivery. Their expertise and background were reflected, at times, in the confidence with which they spoke about health, accessing health care, and criticisms about the health-care system.

Two members of the Experts group grappled with serious health challenges. They were diabetic, one recently diagnosed. The Experts had the most robust discussion about how health barriers are related to racial and gender inequalities. They, like many groups, also stated that women are often doing too much as well as playing so many different roles in society that it interferes with their ability to keep themselves healthy. Also like other groups, they expressed that women tend to minimize their health concerns and put their own needs behind those of others. They felt that women have a lack of support in their households for keeping themselves healthy and often delay seeing a doctor. In addition, they expressed that women sometimes will minimize pain or health ailments and delay seeing a doctor. As one participant shares:

EXPERTS1: I think women are especially good at [thinking] this is going to be alright; I'll just wait on it. And I've seen that have really bad consequences, so I'm always saying, [if] it's a problem you should probably go get somebody to look at that.

EXPERTS2: It's grown! [All laugh a little]

EXPERTS1: But I think it's something that women especially are like, "Oh, it'll be fine, it's a cough today but it'll be alright," those kinds of things.

The Experts, similar to the other mother groups, had health insurance and access to primary care doctors and health-care specialists. The impact of race on health-care services as a topic of conversation emerged organically in this group. They especially talked about providers. Although several of the women in the group have African American doctors, they tended to be especially critical of them. Conversely, several women mentioned double-checking or getting a second opinion about a serious health matter if their doctor was not Black. Their conversation also addressed concerns about how Black women's bodies are perceived by doctors and the need for Black women to pay attention to their health and take it seriously. One of the health educators shared her surprise and frustration that the African American women she comes into contact with lack a basic knowledge about their bodies:

EXPERTS1: I ran a project where we went into churches and I just talked, I mean I thought I was gonna spend; you know, ten minutes on anatomy, female juvenile anatomy. And say oh I'll just go like ten seconds, this is this, this is that, and two hours later these women are asking me questions about what's that, oh, that was there?! Oh, just a basic knowledge of self that was lacking in these 25 adult African American women. I'm like, these women are . . . ! I mean, I really thought I would go really quick over it. And, I had this big drawing that was kind of embarrassing because it was a huge vagina, and you have to do that.

This comment led to a discussion of the ways that the group felt the culture inhibited African American women gaining knowledge about their bodies:

EXPERTS4: Yeah, that's what I was thinking, because it's not just in the health-care system but somewhere it seems like we've lost, you know, sort of the ability to take care of ourselves in a certain way, you know, things that I don't know, I think maybe the educational system or something might be more to blame. I mean now doctors obviously have to be involved because that's their job. But just the basic stuff, why don't people know their anatomy?

They also voiced their perception that African American women may delay getting health news if they think that the news is going to be negative.

The Experts were aware of their daughters' health needs. HIV/AIDS was brought up and discussed in depth by one person when talking about the health challenges their daughters face. But, what takes center stage in their concerns about their daughters' health is helping their daughters to manage a healthy weight and concerns about obesity. As will be discussed in chapter 2, the majority of all the mothers, across groups, worry about school lunches and the influence of junk food, strive to offer their children healthy food choices at home, and try to model for them in particular what they consider a healthy diet (e.g., low sugar, low salt, lots of vegetables).

Unlike other groups where the contrast is much sharper, the Experts group is split almost evenly, with some mothers stating they had good communication about sexuality with their mothers and others saying they had little to none. Experts conveyed the most ease in talking with their daughters about sexual health and voiced the least number of regrets about their own sexual experiences. They expressed the most ease at disclosing important information to their daughters about sexuality. Below is a telling response from one of the members of the group. She expressed her disagreement with other parents at her daughter's school who were leery of sex education being taught in public schools. If anything, she wanted more discussion and was glad for the school's initiative on sexual education.

EXPERTS1: When my daughter took sex-ed in fifth grade I went to a parent meeting and all the parents were like mmm, y 'all don't have to discuss that, don't tell them that, and my daughter was like oh god, she's going in there, she's ready! I wanna know, because I want to know what to talk about at home, I'm excited. So as we sit in the meeting and a bunch of African American parents they were just sitting back watching but the white parents were going, no you're not teaching my child that, you're not going to discuss that, Johnny doesn't need to know all that right now, Susie just needs to know the basics, you know . . . And I'm sitting there going, you can't raise them like that because that's not going work.

The Experts' daughters are slightly younger (12–14), than several of the other groups, so while these mothers are open in certain ways about sexuality, their confidence is not as helpful in imagining what difficulties their daughters may face, as I will demonstrate in chapter 4. They have more challenges imagining and anticipating how their daughters are navigating their bodies. And, as I discuss in chapter 5, their confidence and professional expertise in some cases may distance their daughters from sharing certain kinds of information with their own mothers.

The Transitioners

Transitioners were in a place of change and discovery and grappled with many seismic shifts in their lives, especially as it related to their health. These women talked openly about their struggles with health. Navigating and coming to terms with their new landscape was a worldview that also reflected how they thought about the changes their daughters faced.

There are a few significant differences between the Transitioners group and other groups. Two of the members knew each other previously, which was different than the other groups. Unlike the other groups, two women dominated much of the discussion (not the women that knew each other) and framed their comments in absolute ways (e.g., always, never). They as a group tended to move between biological and religious explanations in describing their understanding of their daughters' behavior (e.g., "she got the wild gene from her father's side of the family"). The composition of this group also differed from others in that one woman was a grandmother raising her granddaughter. Similar to other groups, a person in this group also identified herself as a single parent.

Two of the participants had acute health issues that were discussed. One of the two participants, capturing the feeling of being overwhelmed by her health and the changes that adjusting to this status required, said, "I have all the health problems that you can name." They, like several groups including Experts and Nostalgics, remarked on the challenges that women face in staying healthy. As one member remarked, "I'm efficient in my job, but not my health." This group found common ground discussing that many of their families (especially female members) struggled with diabetes. A salient portion of the conversation included the challenges of dieting, eating healthy, and cooking. They offered cooking ideas and health tips (e.g., eating fruit as a type of snack) to each other. Many were in the process of trying new ways of treating health conditions through nutrition. The Transitioners, like the Experts, discussed the interplay of race and gender on one's experience of health. On the topic of doctors, however, gender mattered more than race. Many of them were divided on the importance of the race of a physician. They differed from the Experts in thinking that having a provider of one's own racial and/or ethnic background was important in terms of possible shared experiences.

They spent much of their time wrestling with the question: What's the biggest health risk that your daughter faces? They were passionately divided between peer pressure and STDs (generally). HIV/AIDS as a potential threat to their daughters' health was also mentioned. As will be explored in chapter 4, many mothers in this group felt that peer pressure could lead their daughters into situations that could have negative consequences.

One of the most intense and revealing moments in all the groups was how the mothers reflected on the question: How would you like your daughter's first kiss to go? In the Transitioners, talking about kissing got them to reflect on what they knew and did not know about their daughters. In discussions of sexual health, they talked of wishing to stress feelings of love and romance and wanted to shy away from the mechanics (as we'll see in chapter 5, most of the daughters, across all the groups, were actually more interested in the mechanics). They wanted to find practical and pragmatic ways to support their daughters in navigating the challenges of young womanhood. In discussing their daughters' sexuality they, like the Revealers discussed below, tended to focus on the moral character of girls, especially those who in their opinion dressed provocatively. There was a lengthy discussion on the clothing choices of their daughters and peers.

The Transitioners talked to each other about the challenges they faced in communicating with their daughters about sexual health. This group, like the Experts, was evenly split in having had some positive conversations with their mothers about sexuality. One of the mothers disclosed that she knew that her daughter had already had sexual relations. The mother was a single parent (and had also been a young mother, having a child at 15) and was the most vocal about needing support and help in dealing with her daughter's evolution from girl to woman. She was also the most vocal individual among all the groups to talk about relying on prayer and the church when feeling stressed. She connected young womanhood to ideas about God and religion:

> Well, I always told my daughter that it's the way you carry yourself, you know what I'm saying? You want to be what God created you to be. This God needs a little girl, needs teenagers and needs a young lady. And, that's the way you're supposed to carry yourself.

Two strategies that these mothers used to discover information about their daughters was searching their daughters' bedrooms and also confirming their daughters' virginity through medical appointments. Their strategies of control were similar to The Strategists, discussed below. In a set of contradictory explanations, they justified their actions by indicating that they were overall more open with their daughters about sexuality than their mothers were with them. The impact of these decisions will be discussed in chapter 4 and chapter 5.

The Revealers

This group's discussion and worldview was defined by the importance of intimacy and disclosure across several members' lives. Intimacy was a characteristic of the group that, like the Transitioners, they tended to share openly. Substantively, their narrative tension and weight came from their thoughts on disclosure on multiple levels of their lives: disclosure and trust of their doctors and health-care providers, what to disclose to daughters, and ongoing levels of disclosure to their own mothers about their lives. Disclosure about their personal failures was also an important defining feature of this group. They also disclosed to each other things that might not have ever been revealed before, including difficult sexual experiences.

Although the focus group began in a lighthearted way and with easygoing energy, it built and gathered an intensity that was unique across the groups. The emotional dynamics and expressiveness of this group was different than the others. It was more emotionally fraught as it dealt more explicitly with grief and reflection. The women in this group both consoled and counseled each other, specifically about the challenges of mother and daughter communication. They ended in a very rich conversational space that touched on power in heterosexual relationships, unlike other groups. Like the Experts, there was one health educator in this group.

Revealers expressed the strongest and most vocal dissatisfaction with their health care and health providers. Although this was the case, ironically, they also most often espoused what can be characterized as a neoliberal understanding of health. They, like the Nostalgics, tend to stress the importance of individual responsibility for health more so than the other groups. I explore this tension further in chapter 2. Although many of them stated that the race of the doctor did not matter, like the Transitioners, there were instances in which they perceived that they were treated differently by Black doctors than by white doctors. Revealers, like the majority of groups, saw the main risks to their daughters' health as caused by obesity, diabetes, and cancer. One person mentioned the threat of STDs and vaguely alluded to HIV.

While there is a focus in all the mother groups about wanting to convey the importance of being an African American young woman and possessing high self-esteem, this is most clearly expressed by the Revealers. Like the Strategists, the Revealers were one of the more proactive groups that had already developed a variety of ways to celebrate their daughters moving into young womanhood; several of them had held "period parties" and made time to mark the passage of girlhood by spending additional time with their daughters in special ways (as defined by them and they daughters). They were interested in discovering additional ways to support their daughters in this transition.

Dating is something the Revealers have discussed at least once with their daughters. In their discussion of mother and daughter communication, they referred to and engaged more popular culture references than other groups and critiqued its depictions of ideal romance. Several of the women made it known that they were frequent church attendees or were active in a church. Several in the group, including a health educator, admitted to struggling with traditional church definitions about love and sexuality and how to communicate that to their daughters without a concomitant feeling of shame. This tension created a place for the participants to reflect on their own beliefs and values. The health educator reflects:

> But I really want to be able to talk with her about what love really is in relation to having sex and be able to have it make sense to her so when she does fall in love, she won't feel guilty. It all comes from something in church that you're made to feel guilty. And I say to my daughter, "I don't want you to see sex as something nasty. It can be something beautiful." And I wish I knew how to communicate that.

All the Revealers grew up in homes where it was taboo to talk about sexual health issues. They uniformly expressed that they were not given helpful or satisfactory knowledge about sexuality and sexual health from their mothers. Unlike the Experts, however, half the group wanted to withhold the stories from their daughters about things they were ashamed of. They traded with each other many of their own personal stories about virginity and early sexual contact. There was a tension that arose for some of the women between wanting to offer up their experiences and their desire to have their daughters abstain from sexual practices. One mother stood out in talking to her daughter in concrete terms about her first sexual experience as a young woman and her difficulties as a single parent. Her discussion redirected the group and contributed tension and a contrast in the group as the other mothers stressed abstinence.

The Nostalgics

The Experts expressed complete confidence, the Transitioners mostly talked about change, the Revealers sought intimacy through disclosure, the Nostalgics' group narrative revolved around keeping calm, seeing themselves as positive influences, and relying on ideas from what has worked for other generations related to mother and daughter communication. The Nostalgics were guided by their sense of personal and family history, and this shaped their approaches to their communication and understanding of their daughters' health. They actively sought out connection and yearned for mother and daughter time. What was striking about their family history was that most of the mothers in this group had mothers and even grandmothers who were alive and physically active.

Health was a priority to these moms for themselves and also for their daughters. One of the mothers revealed she has a chronic health condition. They focused on the challenges of getting their children to eat healthier at home and at school (like the Transitioners and Experts). Their concerns about their daughters' health, like the other groups, also revolved around weight and diet. The Nostalgics emphasized a level of individual responsibility for health, often framing their language about health in terms of choice (similar to the Revealers). Their narratives reveal contradictions as they also discussed many concerns they have about living in conditions where one does not exercise complete control over one's environment (e.g., safe housing) and how that lack of control affects their and others' health. One respondent says:

> I think it's a choice, you know. What makes a woman healthy is having access to either the positive, the choice to be positive, to be in control, the knowledge to sustain your body or at least even the knowledge to know what you should do. Even if you don't do it, at least accept the information and some feeling of living in an environment that is safe and comfortable, free of danger and having at least enough sense of control to be able to make the choices. Because I think there's health and then there's existing. And when I think of what makes a woman healthy, I think of choices.

They also stressed the importance of dealing with various demands of work, children, and partners, and emphasized the need for women to create "me time," and to not just go on autopilot to meet others' demands and "give yourself away."

Like the Transitioners and Revealers, the Nostalgics as a group also had very little sexual health information growing up and wanted to keep the lines of communication open between themselves and their daughters. In a dramatic and powerful moment in the group, one mother shared that she was 13 when she had her first sexual experience and that this experience compels her to want something more for her daughter. In the discussions of teen pregnancy, another mother shared that she had become pregnant at 19.

Similar to other mothers' groups including Revealers, the Nostalgics were worried about peer pressure, which translated into a concern about how other girls might influence their daughters. They expressed a strong desire to keep the lines of communication open and not "freak out" over what daughters might express. As the respondent below notes:

> So, I just try to keep the lines of communication open and hope that she'll never be afraid, ashamed or whatever to talk to me about anything. I try to constantly tell her that there's no subject we can't talk about. "There's no question you can't ask me. There's not anything! Trust me, I may not agree with it. I may not be happy about it. But there is nothing that you can't come to me with because I'm going to tell you the truth. And sometimes your friends don't know. So, they're only going to tell you what they know or what they think they know which is not going to always be the truth. But if you come to me, you'll know you'll get the truth. So, please come to me first." I always can keep that line of communication open; which right now it appears to be that way. I wouldn't think she would withhold anything from me right now. I don't know. But that scares me, if and when that time comes or when that line is crossed, will I know? Will I be able to break that shell again? How will I handle it? That's scary because there's so much out there for them to deal with as children.

Mothers identified the fear that their daughters may have in coming to talk with them as a barrier to communication, as this respondent conveys:

> I just want to be there as a resource for her in terms of managing deep things. Like I don't want her to be so afraid of coming to me about something, that she goes and does stuff and then we have permanent repercussions from that, right? And so that means that I try not to get all bent out of shape and I try not to get all crazy and excited. And I try not to threaten her and I try not to, you know, create all these situations where, you know, she's making desperate decisions without me or without somebody.

They did not possess the same confidence that characterizes the Experts, but they were also not upset or troubled as the Revealers were about their daughters' progression into young womanhood. This might stem from the ways in which they understood young womanhood. They had one of the longest and most in-depth discussions about young womanhood, labeling it as a volatile time of transition. They, like the Transitioners, had a spirited conversation about strategies they use with their daughters to check up on them and make sure they are staying out of trouble. They shared tips and ideas and commended each other on some of those strategies. They had frank conversations about oral sex, anal sex, and the kinds of sexual norms their daughters are exposed to. They also had an extended discussion similar to the Transitioners that expressed their worries about the normalcy of teen pregnancy in high schools. One of the mothers who disagreed with the group's characterization of teenage mothers dropped out of this thread of the conversation.

The Strategists

The worldview that defines the Strategists is their emphasis on protecting, defending, and guarding against a variety of issues (e.g., relationship violence), related to their and their daughters' health and well-being. They had some of the same concerns as Revealers and Nostalgics; however, they saw many more threats than these groups and wondered if they have the capacity to meet them. They also expressed more worry than other mothers about the effectiveness of their communication skills and how they impacted their daughters. They intensely discussed many strategies that involve researching and warding off against threats to their daughters' well-being. They see themselves as having to defend their daughters against other boys' advances and what I call "gendered peer pressure." One of the mothers was dealing with an adolescent daughter who had already borne a child (that daughter is in the corresponding daughters' focus group).

Like the Revealers, the Strategist mothers were also very dissatisfied with the health care they received. They discussed lengthy wait times and unsatisfactory doctor treatment. They often did not feel that their needs were met by medical providers. One woman who was a cancer survivor counseled the others and said that the only way they could deal with a negative health situation is by stressing the need to get a "high amount of information." They also talked at length about their battles with diabetes and breast cancer. This extends to the way they discussed their health; they were worried about being used as "guinea pigs" in research and took drastic steps to find different doctors if they felt this way.

TABLE 1.1. Mothers

Mothers	Experts	Transitioners
Worldview	Expressed a confident and optimistic mindset. Stressed expertise and assuredness about their communication with daughters about health.	They were in the midst of navigating major life changes, often related to their health. They stressed the importance of adaptation.
Conversation Flow	This group is characterized by high energy and direct responses. They did not engage in long pauses, nor were there times where they were unwilling to speak. They often asked each other questions.	This group is characterized by high energy with members who often talked over each other, interrupted each other (and at times the moderator), asked questions, and gave each other advice. Two people sometimes dominated discussion, and framed their comments in absolute ways (i.e., "always" and "never").
Perceptions about Health	They named health barriers related to race and gender. Consensus that women do not prioritize their health needs or, more generally, themselves.	Focused on overcoming personal health challenges. Some members viewed health as a set of individual actions.
Communication with Their Mothers (about sex)	Half of the group reported good communication with mothers about sexuality, the other half had little to no communication with their mothers about sexuality.	They were split in the group, half recalled positive conversations about sexuality with their mothers.
Greatest Concerns about Daughters' Health	Weight was their central concern. HIV is mentioned, but not focused on as major concern.	Teen pregnancy and preventing their daughters from developing a chronic illness.

Similar to the other groups, this group named the things that most concerned them about their daughters' health: a family history of high blood pressure, obesity, diabetes, weight and skin issues. The threat of HIV/AIDS is a concern in this group unlike most of the others. Another thread that was relatively unique to this group was a discussion about whether to vaccinate one's child against the Human Papillomavirus (HPV). One of the women in this group wanted to talk more about HPV, but the group was reluctant to do so.

Like the Revealers, the Strategists were almost unanimous in that they did not have anyone, especially mothers, talking to them about sexuality when they were growing up. Most had no sex education, except one who had a mother who was a nurse. Also similar to the Transitioners and Nostalgics, they had spirited disagreements about teen pregnancy.

Several mothers in this group were determined to break some of the patterns that they experienced growing up in terms of health. One mother said:

TABLE 1.1. (*cont.*)

Revealers	Nostalgics	Strategists
How and what to disclose about their lives to others, including doctors, their daughters, and their mothers was of primary importance.	Guided by a sense of personal and family history in their approach to communicating with their daughters. Looked to the past for solutions.	Saw many threats to their daughters' well-being. Emphasized techniques and practices to manage their daughters' transition into young womanhood.
This group is characterized by high energy. There were several expressive outbursts as members discussed topics of grief and regret.	This group was characterized by steady conversation involving the majority of participants. They counseled each other and gave advice. Long and frank discussion about the volatile nature of adolescence for their daughters.	This group was characterized by high energy, intense discussion, and the expression of very strong opinions, especially about teen pregnancy.
They had the highest dissatisfaction about their health care and their health-care providers.	Several members stressed individual responsibility for one's health. They downplayed external health barriers.	They were dissatisfied with health care. Expressed concern about being used as "guinea pigs" in research because of their race and gender.
The majority of mothers grew up in homes in which it was taboo to talk about sexuality.	They did not have open and frank conversations with their mothers about sexuality.	The majority of mothers did not speak with their mothers about sexual issues during adolescence.
Obesity and diabetes.	Diet, maintaining a healthy weight, and the role of peer pressure.	High blood pressure.

You have to know your history to break it and make it better. I think just with us doing this and talking and just knowing how to talk to our daughters, that's breaking the generational curse. When you say your mama didn't talk to you and you talk to your daughter, that's great.

Despite this more optimistic moment in the group, these mothers, like the Transitioners and Nostalgics, discussed using a variety of strategies and techniques to prevent their daughters' interest in or possibility of having sexual contact. These included surveilling girls through siblings, checking on virginity status through doctors' appointments, and exposing daughters to the real-life rigors of caring for a baby. They had a robust conversation about the effectiveness of their communication. Several mothers acknowledged that although they may talk a lot to their daughters, it does not mean that all the information is sinking in or being received in the way they would like it to.

Summary

As depicted in table 1.1, when we look across all the mother focus groups, striking patterns emerge. In terms of their health, most of the mothers struggled with and were challenged by health issues. They were concerned about hereditary issues that run in their family (i.e., colorectal cancer, heart disease, high blood pressure, etc.). There were members in each group who felt ignored and frustrated by the health-care system, and for the Revealers and Strategists, this was a major point of discussion. All the groups were concerned about their daughters' health and had communicated extensively with their daughters about various aspects of health. There was consensus in several groups on the perception that staying healthy for women is difficult to do because of the particular gendered and/or racialized set of social expectations.

They uniformly shared concerns about their daughters' well-being, especially in terms of their weight and concerns with diabetes. As a group, they halfheartedly shared concerns about HIV along with other STDs. The strategies they used for communicating with their daughters, in analysis, reveal many of their fears and worries. Some of this veered into uncomfortable territory, as we will see in successive chapters. They shared histories of illness in their families and their concerns about how that will shape their daughters' lives.

Generationally, in one voice, they shared the same narrative that the majority of them had little to no sexual health education or discussions about intimacy and sexuality during adolescence. If there were discussions with their mothers, it was of a negative variety, as we shall see very convincingly in chapter 4. They believed and portrayed themselves to be different than their mothers and other female relatives. The mothers openly talked about the need for good, clear communication with their daughters, but also engaged in practices that seemingly undermined their stated trust in their daughters' ability to make responsible decisions.

Overall, in reflecting on the transition to young womanhood, mothers in the majority of the groups expressed concern, challenge, and confusion regarding how to think about how their daughters were making their transition. Mothers with younger daughters tended to express more excitement at the prospects of stewarding daughters through young womanhood. Other mothers struggled to comprehend the changes. Conversation on themes of young womanhood often led to reflections on their own entry into being young women, which was fraught with challenges, as we shall explore more fully in chapter 4.

We have had a look at the mothers and their defining worldviews. Who are the daughters? Who are the groups of girls that made their way into the rooms and shared their perceptions? They ranged from age 12 to age 18, but most girls were around 14 years old. They were lively for the most part, not shy, and shared their thoughts and feelings freely with the moderators.

Daughters

The Romantics

CORRESPONDING MOTHERS' GROUP: THE NOSTALGICS

The Romantics used direct, straightforward language in describing their thoughts throughout the interview. They were positive, optimistic, and their worldview was founded on idealism. The girls offered a more romantic view compared to the other groups in thinking about relationships, and this mirrored the positive and contented ways in which they viewed the world.

The girls' positive and optimistic views informed the way that they discussed their life experiences, ideas about health, and their transition to young womanhood. They also thought of their mothers as healthy, which as we will see with other groups, was not a common perception. And, although they wanted more from their mothers regarding communication about sexuality, their narratives did not express the same kinds of frustration, conflict, regret, or anger as did the four other groups. This group also had more living grandmothers who were active in their lives and with whom they felt bonded. Grandmothers figured prominently in their lives, and the girls commented on the multiple ways that they learned about health from their grandmothers.

As a group, the Romantics expressed confidence and a generous approach toward themselves and others. When they spoke about health, they used a variety of terms that other groups did not, like self-esteem, mind, body, and spirit. They categorically thought of themselves as healthy, though noted some of the same challenges about staying healthy that characterized the other groups (i.e., exercise and diet). Unlike some of the other daughter groups, they faced no personal health challenges.

Of all the daughter groups, the Romantics expressed the most contentment with their bodies and eating habits. They also stressed that they did not need to be perfect, rejecting a language of *lack and deficit*. These girls however did express their desire to always do better in a given situation and to conceal their challenges from others. Here a participant discusses the tension between being strong, not asking others for help and support, and her relationship with herself:

> Well, I know I'm not really but I'm not very—actually—[pause]. I'm not as comfortable with myself as I should. And I don't show it 'cause, like, a lot of my

friends, they'll have problems and stuff. And I'm always, like, the strongest one out of the group. But I don't never show my problems—I don't ever show that I'm not all, like, I love myself, this kind of thing, like I tell them they should be. So, right now, no. But I don't know, I think—I'm going to start working on that because I can't be telling people to love themselves if I don't always love myself. That just don't make no sense.

For the Romantics, the terms "young woman" and "young womanhood" elicited threads of conversations about everything from employing time management strategies to taking more responsibility for themselves. They did not express a consistent or uniform definition about the boundaries that define being a young woman. When and what determines the kinds of signals that welcome them into young womanhood was neither uniform nor agreed on, as these two participants reflect on what they have been told about what signals a transition from girl to woman:

ROMANTICS1: My aunt, my mom, everybody . . . They're like you start your womanhood when you start your period. I was like "OK."

ROMANTICS2: But to my great-grandmother it's when you know how to cook a whole Thanksgiving dinner! [Laughter] I'm dead serious. She's been teaching me for 13 years. And I am not a woman to her. I'm still an infant child because I will burn the turkey. So, yeah.

The girls' relationship and communication with their mothers were characterized mostly in positive terms. The majority of mothers had communicated about their daughters' periods, and some were in the process of talking about sexuality (mostly what not to do). Daughters relied some on mothers for health advice but not primarily for many important issues. When faced with a tough decision, they were more likely to talk to other people instead of their mothers (e.g., aunts). This was not necessarily considered a negative thing like it was for the Distrusters, who we will meet shortly. The Distrusters often felt disrespected by their mothers and therefore avoided communicating with them, whereas the Romantics simply had a preference for talking to godmothers, older sisters, and grandmothers.

Regarding conversations about intimacy and sexuality, only one girl in this focus group had received zero communication about sexuality from her mother. She mentioned that her dad and grandmother had been instrumental in talking with her about sexual issues.

ROMANTICS3: My mom hasn't ever told me anything. My dad, he's told me about dates and stuff. But he hasn't really gotten to it. But my grandmother, she said always make sure that you find the key to your heart before you open the door.

Ohhh! Someone shouts [Cross-talk, girls respond enthusiastically]

ROMANTICS2: I like that. [Others agree]

ROMANTICS3: She's so good.

[Continued cross-talk—very animated]

This phrasing of "find the key to your heart" became a defining moment in the conversation that participants repeatedly referenced. One girl returned to this idea and said, "I like what you said about the key." They used the metaphor of the key to talk about decision making generally, and how to make decisions about relationships in particular. They used this to talk about the difference they perceived between sex and intimacy—making decisions based just on someone's looks or peer pressure as opposed to genuine feelings.

Concerns about pregnancy were on the girls' minds and emerged in the conversation through what they heard, but also from their access to media, including watching "baby shows." The girls were equally intrigued, disgusted, and worried about childbirth and "the painful parts." Sometimes watching shows at school or home triggered a conversation with a mother about childbirth, as one participant notes:

> I've had conversations with my mother a lot about childbirth. I keep asking her questions from it. But she doesn't always respond.
>
> . . . But it's like some of parts of the show (about being pregnant and having a baby) make me not want to get pregnant. But they (the young women in the reality show) would look forward to it . . . and then some other parts of it—oh, my God! It's just like an evil, painful part.

Sometimes when a daughter posed questions to her mother, the exchange might lead to a longer conversation, but that did not always guarantee that the girl's questions were fully answered. An observation from this focus group was that, although the girls overall expressed trust and connection to their mothers and had a more romantic view about relationships, they were simultaneously eager to discuss more details about sexuality. This was true of other daughter groups, too.

The Equalizers

CORRESPONDING MOTHERS' GROUP: THE EXPERTS

The Equalizers' worldview encompassed recognizing gendered inequality in particular and discussing it as it manifested in the double standards of their lives. They viewed the world where girls are often on the losing end of the social hierarchy and talked about how that affected them. These were among the defining moments of the conversation. Interestingly, although the Equalizers were daughters of the Experts, a group with a lot of professional knowledge and discussion of health, their expertise did not always seem to correspond to the daughters' perceptions and experiences of health. They struggled more than the other groups with defining what health meant to them. That part of the conversation was marked with nervous laughter and an admission by one of the girls that she eats "when she's bored." Unlike the Romantics, health was a sterile and hygienic affair for the Equalizers. For some, health was being clean and taking a bath regularly. They tended not to think of themselves as healthy.

Most Equalizers viewed their mothers as healthy. However, several were concerned about their mothers' mental health, especially their stress levels:

EQUALIZERS1: I don't think that my mom is really happy anymore and it makes me really sad. 'Cause I mean she has two sisters and her dad died when I was six. And it was like really hard times for her and then her stepmom died and then um, I don't remember when her stepmom died; it was maybe when I was eight. And then earlier this year her mom died and ever since then she's been really down and been staying at work really really late and when she comes home then she goes on the computer to finish what she didn't finish at work. She goes in early [to work] and then doesn't go to sleep 'til one [a.m.]. And when you're like around her she seems sort of down and you look at her and she like smiles and tries to make it seem like everything's fine but I just feel like it's not, and I wish I knew what to do.

This comment elicited a longer comment from another member who recounted her grandparents' divorce after 36 years and the effect this has had on her mother who, the daughter says, has been "upset" because of the challenges this presents for her.

EQUALIZERS2: My mom, she doesn't get any sleep anymore because it's like, my grandma will call and she'll start fussing about something that my grandpa did and my grandpa will call and start fussing about something my grandmother did and my mother's like, "I really can't deal with the stress."

My mom's the oldest so the younger kids really look up to her so when they see my mom she'll try to hide it, but then sometimes she's just, doesn't want to talk to anybody.

My mom, she has like kidney problems, stuff like that, so just to see her down it just makes my whole day just . . . that's how I feel, like she's unhappy.

The Equalizers tended to be more father-centered than the other groups—relying on their dads for advice for many aspects of life. Their relationship with their mothers in terms of communication about health and sexuality was strained and contentious. They expressed very strong feelings that school was a better place to find out about things related to sexuality, which is distinctive from the other groups.

The Equalizers offered language about the names boys use for girls and to describe sex. This led into a discussion about the different ways that boys and girls are perceived about their sexuality. This thread of conversation was a defining one in the group.

EQUALIZER82: I think to females it's more sacred, but to boys it's just like something . . . and I feel like, like people may have, this is my problem, like I feel like people say like females should be put here [in a box] but what about boys? I feel like they put a lot on women about sex and stuff, but not a lot on men. Like they're always like, a female is a ho, but what about a boy? Why is he not a ho?

There was agreement in the group with Equalizer2's observation about girls and boys being treated in different ways. In the midst of this agreement, she goes on to elaborate and is joined in the discussion by another participant:

EQUALIZERS2: I remember my grandma like telling me like she was like telling me stories about her old life. She was like, "I didn't have sex 'til I was married." And my grandma got married when she was 21. Well these days girls don't really do that because they feel like they have to give it up to people to make them feel like they're loved.

EQUALIZERS3: A lot of boys make girls feel like it's the right thing to do, you're supposed to do it and if this is not done you're just like an outcast. I mean it hits especially once you get to high school. People are just like you know, you ain't done it yet? What's wrong with you? You ain't like the rest of us. And, a lot of girls do it just to get attention.

The Equalizers expressed strong emotions throughout the focus group about how boys and girls are treated differently. While the Equalizers pointed to the challenges and unfair burden that girls carry, they also tended to blame girls for certain kinds of behavior (including wearing revealing clothes). This finding was interesting and surprising, as their mothers were the least likely of all the mother groups to discuss girls' attire. As I will explore more fully in chapter 5, I would argue that the girls' hostility toward other girls can be interpreted as frustration within a larger cultural system that encourages them to devalue girls. Their attitudes inform a type of respectability politics, one that is manifested in discussions scrutinizing some girls' dress and what they consider transgressive behavior.

The Loners

Corresponding Mothers' Group: The Revealers

The Loners are distinctive among the daughters' groups in a variety of ways. Their narratives were marked throughout by anger and frustration and they were generally a low-energy group. They were more suspicious of adults as a whole in comparison to the other groups. Their worldview was one of disconnection. The dominant image that comes through is the negative experience of being adrift, alone, and without a lot of support. They were disconnected from many people, but especially their mothers; they did not relate to or identify with them. This disconnected worldview created a context for them to see themselves as less interdependent than others and to cast themselves as rebels.

Strikingly, the girls of the Loners group unanimously did not define themselves as healthy. Health for them was a blank slate; few feelings or emotions were involved in how they talked about their personal health. They were split on whether their mothers were healthy, and the instances when they talked about their mothers not being healthy was also usually related to eating fast food or junk food.

The girls' feeling suspicious and seeing themselves pitted against the world alone spills over into how they talked about their health experiences. They voiced negative opinions about doctors. One participant had a very strong opinion about doctors because of a negative experience she perceived in how her grandfather was treated.

The Loners spent time talking about the context of communication between them and their mothers. Communication with mothers was particularly poor in this group. One girl had a clear conflict with her mother and used extreme language to describe the ways in which they did not get along.

Their corresponding mother group was the Revealers, and similar to daughters in other groups, the Loner daughters felt penalized and scrutinized for asking questions about sexuality. Once they began digging into this topic, they connected with each other. These girls were more willing to talk freely about challenges they faced, and they gave each other advice. The girls talked to each other about the difference between sex and intimacy. There was disagreement among them, and they had many questions. The primary things this group wanted to learn about becoming a woman included learning about relationships, how to be successful without a man, and what it means to experience independence. In answering the question, "Is there anything that you wanted to talk about or ask your mother about becoming a woman that you haven't yet?" the daughters recounted examples of previous attempts at communication with their mothers that were stilted or that resulted in feelings of increased scrutiny:

LONERS1: I wanted to ask her something, but if I ask her she would probably think that I was about to go have sex. 'Cause one time I asked her like could you get pregnant if you had sex in the pool. And then she was like, "Well, you went to the pool today." I said "What?" [Laughter from all] I was like "No!" And then like I wanted to ask her about, you know how people talk about when you first do it, like it's supposed to hurt or whatever. I wanted to ask her because I was thinking about doing it or whatever. But I didn't want her to know. I just wanted to see what she was going to say. But I didn't ever ask her because I knew she would be like "Now, you can't go to this party and that 'cause you'll probably decide to have sex."

LONERS2 (INTERRUPTS): [Asks rhetorical question about why parents don't see things the way young people do] Like, OK, if you don't talk to your child about certain things, especially stuff like sex or drugs, if you do not talk to your child, then they got to go get information from somewhere else, nine times out of ten they will go and they will do it just because they don't feel open to go talk to their parents about stuff. And that's how I feel now. I feel like "OK, well, if you can't talk to me about it, I'll find out from somebody else." When I find out from somebody else, it's like one of my peers and they're telling you "Oh, it's good!"

This provides an important perspective, as will be discussed in later chapters. The mothers across the groups perceived their communication as effective, direct, and different than their own mothers' communication. In many cases across groups, the daughters had their own filters that suggest otherwise.

One Loner talked about having watched Lifetime movies with her mother, which she enjoyed until her mother badgered her to talk about issues of sex and intimacy to the point where the mother became frustrated and the daughter became tired. The frequent disconnect between the mothers' and daughters' perceptions of the timing of communication about sexuality will be explored in chapters 4 and 5.

The Moderates

CORRESPONDING MOTHERS' GROUP: THE STRATEGISTS

There seems to exist in just about any typology a group that straddles the middle. This is true of the Moderates group. Their narratives were not delineated by strong feelings or long discussions about either their or their mothers' health or communication about sexuality. They took an informed basic approach to all of these topics. Things that made them more distinctive were that, like the Romantics, they had grandmothers they consulted and were close to. Questions about sexuality, culture, and the media were the most animating and most noteworthy topics of conversation. This is also the only group where a discussion of social media figured prominently. Moderates had the most age diversity among the daughter groups, with ages ranging from 12 to 16. This age range did not detract from the discussion, as the younger girls spoke up frequently.

The Moderates' definitions of health were divided into two categories like the Equalizers: "being clean" and "using hygiene." Like all other groups, food appeared significantly as a main challenge for their health. Several of the girls said they were not as healthy as they would like to be, which echoes the Equalizers and Distrusters. They had extended discussions with their grandmothers about health and used what they described as "old-time remedies," remedies that are not pharmaceutical. In this group compared to the others, money was mentioned prominently in connection with being a young woman. Several of the girls had more responsibility for managing the household budget and understanding finances in a detailed way.

The Moderates were very media-savvy and often developed their responses by drawing on current popular culture, including Britney Spears and BET videos as well as documentaries about rape and sexual violence. Without being prompted, they noted the media's influence in shaping girls' experiences of sexuality and how they should act with boys. In terms of mother and daughter communication about sexuality, this group was split. Some would prefer not to talk with their mothers about these issues and others indicated that they were open to such conversation.

Sexual orientation was discussed at length in this focus group, also marking it as distinctive from the other groups. One girl came out, identifying as lesbian, at the end of the focus group and talked about her challenges in school with peers and her parents.

The Distrusters

CORRESPONDING MOTHERS' GROUP: THE TRANSITIONERS

The Distrusters spent most of their time expressing suspicion, concern, and distrust toward two groups—parents and doctors. There was a pervasive framing that the world of adults did not have their best interests at heart. One important area of narrative energy was the depth of discussion surrounding negative responses to doctors. This group went the most in-depth about negative responses to doctors, with the majority expressing challenges in their dealings with them. The Loners held a general distrust of doctors, but the Distrusters had several negative experiences. The Distrusters, like the Moderates, were also heavy media consumers and extracted some of their ideas from media. Their patterns of communication with people looked much more like a mosaic than the other groups. They conversed with fathers and grandmothers and sometimes with mothers. Another unique feature of this group was that one of the daughters was already a mother.

As I discuss in the last section of the chapter, the theme of respect figured prominently across the groups. This group in particular felt disrespected from mothers and other adult figures. They stated that the reason they didn't confide in their mothers often was because their trust had been violated more than once. Instead, they often sought out sisters, aunts, and other close female relatives for discussions about issues of importance to them.

They defined themselves as being "in the middle" and "in between" when it came to their health. One girl had a serious heart condition. They framed their health challenges in similar ways to other groups. They did not exercise often and enjoyed watching many hours of television. To stay healthy, they liked to ride bikes, walk, and dance. The barriers to being healthy were framed as laziness, sleeping, eating junk food, and being influenced by "the devil." Girls in the Distrusters group expressed some concern that going outside to exercise could lead to a threat or a confrontation. The mother in this group of Distrusters had a son that was a toddler; she expressed being unable to be more active because she had a child, which prevented her from doing things because "I just stay in and watch him."

Talk in this group heated up when they discussed their view of boyfriends and their responsibilities toward them. The responses created more dynamic interaction between them. One participant said to watch out for boys looking "for relations not a relationship."

Like Equalizers, Distrusters posed questions about fairness and girls having negative reputations. Threaded through some of their discussions was blaming girls for perceived promiscuity, including "going out with every dude they see" or, more incitingly, "some girls will do the whole squad." The discussion of being young women introduced the use of the Internet as a resource. The Distrusters are intentional about going on the Internet to search for concepts related to being a young woman; they mentioned specific websites they use, including young-teens.com. They, more than the Moderates, relied on the Internet for resources.

Their communication about sexual health with mothers focused on their knowing about their periods, but little else. One girl indicated that her father had initiated the "boyfriend conversation," but nothing more intimate than that. Another participant declared, "My mom never really talked to me

TABLE 1.2. Daughters

Daughters	Romantics	Loners
Worldview	Upbeat and positive orientation. Idealistic.	Detached. Disconnected from peers and family.
Conversation Flow	Conversation flowed easily.	Chaotic at times. Girls joked with each other and moderator, sometimes did not seem to take themselves seriously. Moved in and out of intense conversation.
Perceptions of Health	Connected to self-esteem and confidence. They unanimously described themselves as healthy. Half described their mothers as healthy.	They unanimously defined themselves as unhealthy. Members of the group were split on whether their mothers were healthy.
Communication with Their Mothers (about sex)	Relied on others for information about sex but stressed that they could talk with their mothers. Several rely on others for info about sex and intimacy—but stressed that they could talk with their mothers.	They did not rely on mothers for information about sex.
Miscellaneous	They have more living grandmothers than other groups.	Daughters discussed being punished for asking questions about sexuality.

about sex. I learned on my own." What is striking about their answers to and discussion about the body, health, and particularly sexuality, is that Distrusters were high media and Internet users, but seemingly possessed low sexual knowledge. The Moderates, on the other hand, possessed both high media interest and knowledge of their bodies. Strikingly, the only young woman in this group to have a child seemed to know a little more about the mechanics of sex than the other girls. They were getting some information from others, but most often from TV and particularly videos. They overall had less critical opinions of the how the media shaped their preferences compared to other users in the Moderate and Equalizer groups.

TABLE 1.2. (*cont.*)

Moderates	Equalizers	Distrusters
Media savvy and often developed their responses by drawing on popular cultural references.	Concerns about gender equality were central.	Suspicious of authority figures (e.g., parents and doctors) and sometimes peers.
Widest spread of ages of girls in any group. Group members took about ten minutes to warm up. After that time, the conversation was steady.	Strong and steady.	Although one of the smaller groups in size, members shared freely.
Eating healthy food was a main challenge. Several of the girls said they were not as healthy as they would like to be.	Most did not think of themselves as healthy.	Dissatisfied with the health care they experienced. Described themselves in the middle with their health.
The group was split. Some would prefer not to talk with their mothers about sex and others indicated that they were open.	Strained dynamic with the girls and their mothers. Only one of the girls has had a conversation about sex with her mother.	Aunts and sisters play an important role as conveyers of knowledge about sexuality. Most had not had substantive conversations with mothers about sex and intimacy.
In this group compared to others, money came up significantly as being connected to young womanhood. Several of the girls shoulder more responsibility for managing the household budget and understanding finances compared to other groups. One girl identified as lesbian at the end of the focus group.	Group members expressed strong feelings that school was a better place (than home) to find things out about sexuality (from teachers and counselors), which is distinctive from the other groups.	There is a young mother in this group.

Becoming a Young Woman

Based on group consensus, young womanhood was viewed as a transitional period between childhood and becoming a mature woman. Young womanhood involves the development of physical, emotional, and mental maturity. The girls emphasized the importance of being responsible for their decisions and planning for their future. In addition, they felt it was necessary to develop basic survival skills, such as cooking, cleaning, budgeting money, and paying bills. In some cases, the daughters were given new responsibilities by the adults in their lives, even if they did not yet feel ready to take them on.

For the majority of groups, the discussion lingered on the roles and responsibilities that come with being a young woman and the sense of being "in between" one set of expectations and another. The Moderates identified this liminal space they were navigating as being marked by physical changes but also increased responsibilities.

MODERATES1: [on young womanhood] . . . it's like you're not yet to the maturity of being a woman, but you're almost there. Like you've found confidence in yourself, you know what you're about, you know what you want, that kind of thing.

MODERATES2: I'm gonna sound like a big geek when I say this but it's like that [lyric from] Britney Spears song, "I'm not a girl but not yet a woman" [all laugh loudly]. But it's true . . . it's true when like, I don't really go for the song, but like that part of the song, it's true you're not a girl, you're not a little kid anymore, but you're not a woman. You're not like at the full kinda like boom stage, you're right there in transition.

MODERATES3: It's exactly like transition.

[Someone else says this was a good example]

MODERATES4: It's like that line that's like okay I'm this age, so maybe I need to act this age, you know be more mature than I was before.

At this point in the focus group, there was discussion about when young womanhood begins. Later, there is agreement that it starts around the ages of 12 or 13. When the interviewer asked when does it end, several girls said "18, 19," and another said "definitely 20."

Moderates3 clarifies, "I don't think you can really break it down by age . . . once I hit this age then I'm a woman. I think you have to go emotionally like how you are on an emotional level and mentally because you can be as old as you want to be and still act like a little kid. It depends on how you are as a person." Moderates1 went back to the idea that age doesn't solely define what it means to be a young woman. She stressed that when you are a young woman, you do not have to rely on someone else.

The participant who began the discussion with Britney Spears closed out the discussion by ruminating about her own experience of responsibility:

MODERATES2: I agree with actually all of them because like a lot of days like nowadays girls grow up a lot faster than they're supposed to, like me. I'm supposed to be a 15-year-old but I do a lot of the stuff that a 23-year-old do as far as taking care of the bills, making sure everything's done, I do a lot of the stuff that a grown woman's supposed to do, but I do it for the family. You know, that kind of thing, so I think it all depends on the maturity of you and the emotional, also the age.

Some girls experienced the increased responsibility as being stressful. A few terms they used to describe the experience of being a young woman included "being grown," "take care of myself," and "being responsible."

We turn now to physical markers of transition. Some of the girls had not had a specific conversation about menstruation with their mothers, but most had and were aware that this physical change marked a new stage of life. For many girls, menstruation was the very definition of being a young woman, anchored by what they were told by female figures. This comment from a participant in the Romantics group is representative of the majority of comments:

I would say when you become a woman that you get your period. That's what I mean by that. That starts a woman to me. That's all of what my mom told me starts your womanhood. My aunt, my mom, everybody. They're like you start your womanhood when you start your period. I was like "OK."

Health for the daughters was often a mixed picture. The Loners unanimously said they did not define themselves as healthy. Three other groups—the Moderates, the Equalizers, and the Distrusters—were mixed, mostly leaning toward not defining themselves as healthy. Some girls used the language of being "in between." Only in the Romantics group did all of the participants describe themselves as healthy. Overall, the girls blamed themselves for eating junk food and not exercising. Many also did not see their mothers as healthy. Their perceptions of health will be discussed in-depth in chapter 3.

The daughters generally relied on a variety of people besides their mothers for communication about important issues involving health and sexuality. For some groups, as with many of the Loners and Distrusters, this was because of an adversarial and contentious relationship with their mothers. Others drew on a wide network of family, girlfriends, and boyfriends. Another important takeaway that will be explored in chapter 5 is that the majority of the girls did not feel that they had access to adequate communication about sexuality.

The major themes about young womanhood that emerged from the data are those of respect, pressure, and trust.

Respect

Respect is intimately linked with others, though the daughters often present it as being about one's self. Respect is a theme that cuts across the girls' under-standing of themselves as people who will make intimate decisions, especially when it comes to romantic relationships. Every focus group discussed respect in relation to being a young woman: from the very basic statement, "My mom always tells me to respect myself," to the idea of respect functioning as a fundamental mechanism aspect of navigating young womanhood. For these girls, respect was coded through a level of embodiment—how one "carries" oneself was a standard way that girls discussed how they understood what it meant to be treated well in the world. This example from the Loners exemplifies this perspective:

> Well, mama said, like, as you get older, your environment changes as do the people you hang around. Like, you can't hang around these same people. I don't know how to say this but, a lot of stuff about you that has to change. You got to carry yourself in a different way 'cause you're older.

Daughters in the groups are highly attuned to when they do not feel respected in their personal relationships. They have picked up the message that you always want to have respect in relationships.

In the Equalizers, after discussing what their mothers told them about becoming young women, the conversation moved to a discussion of boys and respect quickly emerged:

EQUALIZERS2: How they're supposed to treat you, like my mom always tells me like people will respect you if you respect yourself. So always think of that when you think of a boy. He won't respect you. Like she tells me what I should expect from a boy, so for me, instead of not, thinking less of myself, you know, don't lower my standards, that's what she says.
[Answering a question, the moderator asked: Are boys a topic of discussion? Many answer yes.]

MODERATOR: [Really, okay.] And what are those conversations like?

EQUALIZERS5: She reminds me of what her mother told her . . . she tells me you know, respect yourself and he'll respect you and she's talking about what he should do and how he should treat you. And her thing is that if he just treats you like dirt . . . just some ordinary girl, then it's a problem.

Respect was on these girls' minds as they entered into friendships and other intimate relationships. Respect was also about how you present yourself to the world through behavior and clothing. We hear from the Equalizers again:

EQUALIZERS3: Even girls don't have respect for other females, like you should respect a girl enough not to sit there and stare at her boyfriend. Or not to look her up and down or not to disrespect her, call her a b—, because if girls disrespect each other, this is something I've learned, if girls disrespect each other, then a boy will disrespect you because they feel like if girls are gonna disrespect each other then why can't I do it?

In one exchange, a participant from the Loners group expressed quite strongly not feeling respected by her mother. She had just finished sharing with the interviewer that she "hates it when her mother tells her 'don't have sex.'"

MODERATOR: Well, why do you hate that?

LONERS1: This is why I hate that, because if somebody—and this is just for anything—if somebody keeps telling me not to, "you're not gonna do something," I tend to be like "Oh, so, it must be good if you're keeping something away from me. Or are you telling me that I'm not going to do it like I'm your slave. I understand that you're my mother but you still have to treat me with some respect because you want respect back. And when she tells me "don't have sex," I feel like "Oh, so it must be good if you're trying to keep"—you know what I'm saying? . . .

Well, I tell her, regardless, I appreciate your advice. I mean I tell the truth. I'm sorry. I cannot lie. I say, you know, "Part of being a parent is being a guide to your child. And I appreciate that. But also you have to realize that sooner or later I'm gonna grow up and I'm going to be an adult. And, you know, you're not going to always be there for me. You can give me guidance, but don't push your problems or what you want me to do onto me. You can tell me what you think might be best for me. But don't tell me what I am and I ain't gonna do 'cause I'm still gonna do what I want to do." And that's just being true.

Respect for this participant also looked like being given truthful information and sharing all the options. This participant had a particularly difficult relationship with her mother, but the other girls agreed with the larger sentiment.

Respect emerged quite strongly for this group when we talked about health care. Distrusters talked about losing respect for nurses given what they saw as negative or inferior treatment of their grandparents, as well as in interpersonal relationships and arguments that mothers and daughters had (i.e., you don't respect me).

Pressure

Adolescence is generally a heightened time of experience, as young people encounter and learn to navigate social messages about their appearance, mannerisms, and abilities and how they will act in peer relationships. For some adolescents, this transition is like navigating a high wire, for others it can feel like being on display in a fish bowl, sometimes it feels like both of those situations are happening simultaneously. Many areas of an adolescent's life cause the experience of pressure and stress. Pressure, as a tangible force, reverberated through several aspects of the girls' lives. Girls feel pressure from their peers, their parents, and the media. Pressure as a feeling is connected to managing relationships, financial concerns, and general family issues and for some, the expectations for college.

The sense of being pressured animated discussions in both subtle and overt ways. The daughters also talked about the stress in their lives that resulted from what they considered as undue pressure. The different types of pressure daughters felt tops the list of what many girls most wanted their mothers to understand about the challenges that they faced.

Right before the quote below, this participant in the Equalizers said that she feels "held down" and "restrained" because of the people in her life asking her to do various things, these requests and expectations "stress her out" and she often did not want to do them. She articulated feeling unhappy with herself about not wanting to complete the request and therefore letting family members down.

EQUALIZERS5: I feel actual pressure on me because people are always asking so much from me and I feel like people ask a lot from me just because, well I'm the youngest like in grandchildren and all my other cousins are like failures. Not really failures, but they're . . . Everybody in my family, like my grandma puts a lot of stress on me 'cause she's like well you gotta go to school and you gotta do this and this. I just feel stressed and pressured sometimes, like really stressed out.

Unfortunately, we do not know what the "stuff" is exactly, but from this participant's previous comments, we can infer that a large component of this stress relates to achievement, including applying for things that will provide recognition.

Later in the conversation, another participant offered this understanding about pressure:

EQUALIZERS2: My older cousin just had a baby, she was seventeen and so, one of my cousins dropped out of high school and my boy cousin he's just like whatever, I don't care. And I'm younger than all of them and I had a job this summer. And they didn't have one. I mean, I make better grades than them. My cousin is really smart; I mean she could do anything she wants to do. She wanted to be a cosmetologist, but she's so smart, she made straight A's all through the year she was in high school, until she dropped out. You know, I'm like, why, everybody puts pressure on me because they're like, you're the last one so you know, you have to be better than them—

EQUALIZERS5: —They have hope—

EQUALIZERS2: Yeah you have hope. You know, so I'm like, everyone's like well you got into Reedswell College,[4] wow, beautiful, whatever. So everyone's putting pressure on me now, I feel like I have to make straight A's or if I don't then everyone's going to fuss at me and stuff, so I feel like I have to do this kind of stuff because I have to be better than them and that's how they always treat me, you need to be better than them, so I have a different pressure than y'all, I'm like, they're pushin' me to do better than them. So I guess that's kind of positive pressure but at the same time I feel like they push me too much sometimes.

This participant in the Equalizers is an example of the ways many girls, across groups, would talk about pressure they experienced in dealing with boys:

EQUALIZERS3: I feel stressed out too sometimes but I also feel like it's hard for me to make something of myself out there in the world because it feels like you know, like she says right, because people are trying to put pressure on you and people are telling you, you know, you need to do this and you need to do that and you know if you don't do this you're gonna . . . and also because like a lot of girls put that stereotype on girls so a lot of boys look at you as like you ain't nothing but another ho. I mean I'm not a ho, but people put that out there, people [will] say you know I don't care you are all in that same stereotype.

As stated earlier, this group was highly attuned to the challenges girls face about sexuality and sexual expression relative to boys. In other focus groups, girls talked more about pressure to have intercourse, or to go further sexually than they wanted to with a young man. Girls across all groups believed they faced pressure by young men and that images of girls and women from the media pressure girls to be sexual.

Trust

Communication involves trust. Who are the people the girls trust with important things in their lives? Who do they trust with their health? The girls discussed whom they talk to when important issues arise in their life regarding school, friendships, relationships, and their health. As a whole, the girls had a wide variety of people with whom to communicate about health, sexuality, and other important issues. Strikingly, mothers for many of the groups were in the background. Mothers were often trusted with school matters, but frequently were not their daughters' closest confidantes. Sisters, aunts, cousins, and other female family figures played a role, as did some fathers. Moreover, peers played an important role.

As one respondent said, "Family stuff goes to mom. Any other stuff she won't understand." Across all focus groups, a high number of girls in each group indicated that they did not communicate "important stuff" or questions of intimacy with their mothers first. This was especially true for the following groups: Equalizers, Loners, and Distrusters. In chapter 5, I discuss why these groups may be particularly less invested in talking to their mothers.

This exchange from the Loners about not trusting their mothers highlights an exchange often replicated across groups:

MODERATOR: Who is the first person among your family that you communicate with about important issues?
LONERS1: My cousin.
MODERATOR: Why do you talk to your cousin?
LONERS1: 'Cause I can't trust my mother.

Here are some of the reasons girls noted for why they trusted others about important information across focus groups:

−I trust her [my sister] because she just tells me some of her deepest darkest secrets and she never told my mom. And, I trust her with my deepest darkest secrets.
−I trust my boyfriend because I can tell him how I feel.

–My godmother will want to listen to me more than my mother does.
–A friend will keep a secret if you want her to.
–Well, I have a girl best friend and I have the kind of friends who I've known
  for a long time and I would tell either of them because we both have a
  certain amount of trust.

Mothers work very hard to establish both authority and trust, but that is not always what daughters experience. The reasons for the lack of trust include not feeling listened to, that others did a better job of listening, a belief that their mother couldn't relate or understand the issue being contemplated (especially involving intimate matters), and believing that their mothers would violate their trust. One explanation is that many felt that their mothers would talk to others about something important. For several of the girls, their trust had been violated previously. When they talked about why they did not go to their mothers, it was because mothers violated their trust in other situations.

There was a particularly strongly held opinion that mothers could not be trusted to pass on information to other people in the family. In this example, first from the Distrusters and then the Loners, some of the participants express strong feelings.

MODERATOR: You talk mostly to your aunt. And why your aunt?
DISTRUSTERS2: She doesn't spread anything to my mom. She understands better
    than my mom.
MODERATOR: And why is that? Why do you say that?
DISTRUSTERS2: 'Cause certain stuff I tell my mom she don't understand. She gets mad.
MODERATOR: Can you give an example?
DISTRUSTERS2: Pregnancy and sex. [delivered in a low voice]

MODERATOR: [addressing a particular girl]: Why do you talk to your cousin?
LONERS1: Because I can't trust my mother . . . Like if I tell my mother some-
    thing—if I tell her promise not to tell nobody—she tells somebody!
    [Nods and murmurs of agreement among the girls]

Besides the strong belief by many girls that their mothers would disclose sensitive information, there was also an expressed belief by many girls that their mothers just do not understand. The exchange that follows, from the Moderates, offers important insight into why girls sometimes withhold information from mothers. One of the girls indicated that she would first talk to a cousin about something important.

MODERATES4: Or like somebody my age because there's some stuff that you, that's happened to me that you can't tell your mom 'cause it might upset her or she might not get the picture, so you have to go to a cousin first to go through the whole promise thing, promise not to tell.

MODERATOR: Okay, so and I heard some kind of agreement about wanting to talk to somebody close to your age.

MODERATES3: I actually said my mama instead of somebody that's my age. Me personally, me and my mom have a really close relationship and she's open minded so we don't really have that many problems communication wise so I can go to her.

The conversation continues:

MODERATES1: I think it just depends on what it is. Like, if it's like academic wise, like I got a hundred on my test [I would tell my mother] or if it's like oh I go with this person and this person, I would tell my friend that but I wouldn't tell my mama that because sometimes she doesn't understand. It just depends on what it is. It's like, sometimes like secretly I think your mom don't want to know certain stuff [everyone agrees], I think she just wants you to do your thing and just don't get caught is what I think.

MODERATES2: She be like, oh okay, you can tell me everything!

MODERATES5: Then she'll be like, I can't believe you didn't tell me!

MODERATES3: You can tell them to an extent and then past that point they don't really want to know.

MODERATES1: Sometimes I think you have to tell your mom.

[Moderator encourages Moderates1 to continue and clarify]

MODERATES1: Uh, I think that sometimes you have to tell your mom because sometime it can put kind of a blocker on you guys' relationship. So I think sometimes you have to tell, you might not want to, but sometimes it might make your relationship better, so I think sometimes you got to tell.

This is a moment of importance in the girls' lives as they revealed having questions and concerns about relationships, intimacy, navigating friendships. In this focus group they stood out as unique in reflecting on the reasons and consequences for not telling and consequently trusting their mothers. They also discussed the subtle dance of what to inform mothers about as well as maybe the benefits of not telling.

What might explain this troubling finding? Girls could be uniquely sensitive at this age to ideas about trust, and that may not be as important to mothers or on the radar. As we shall see in chapter 5, for the girls who don't trust their mothers, some significant challenges surface when we examine issues of sexuality and sexual health. Perhaps these groups who have low communication issues are unique. But, given that the majority of daughters do not regularly communicate with their mothers on important issues, it could indicate further problems down the line as they may obtain inaccurate information. The mothers continue to believe that they have effective communication with their daughters. As we shall see in following chapters, how the girls experience, understand, and respond to pressure, trust, and respect shape and influence how they think about their health across multiple domains.

Conclusion

This chapter has provided an introduction to the mother and daughter focus groups. In identifying the characteristics of the groups, I have outlined the perspectives that governed each one that reflects a worldview of the group and group concerns. The worldviews capture their ideas about physical and sexual health. These perspectives help lay the foundation for exploring and understanding the narratives around mothers' communication of health and sexuality. The mothers overall perceived themselves to be knowledgeable, open, and as laying the foundation for effective communication about a variety of health issues. They worked on their health and struggled with diet and exercise. The daughters, in contrast, did not as a whole confide in their mothers for many important matters. We will see how the disjuncture between mothers' and daughters' understandings and tensions shape expectations and understandings for both groups as we look deeply at how these narratives emerge for health and sexuality. There is a recurring way in which they seem to talk "past" each other, resulting in conflicting narratives.

2

Mothers' Health Narratives

This chapter explores African American mothers' concepts of health and well-being, including how they defined and perceived health, how their perceptions of health are tied to their mothers' experiences with health, and how they communicated about their family's history of health to their daughters. Their narratives also reveal their hopes and fears about their daughters' health.

Four themes emerge in the mothers' narratives of health: (1) mothering practices of health, (2) implicit and explicit barriers to health, (3) how race and gender inform their experiences navigating health care, and (4) their perceptions of risk of daughters' health.

Attention to how the focus group participants discuss their mothers' health reveals their mothers' experiences are like their own, rooted in systemic micro- and macro-inequalities marked by gender, race, and class. The intergenerational legacy of seeing chronic health conditions play out in their family, and their mothers' resilience, shape the participants' understanding of health. This "health inheritance" provides insight into aspects of mothers' decision-making processes and communication with their daughters about health.

The participants, like the majority of women in America, are full-time workers and undertake multiple caretaking roles for older (and often sick) parents, children, and spouses or partners. Some of the mothers also faced stressors of job insecurity, lack of access to health care, and the management of chronic health issues (theirs and in a few cases even their daughters'). Every focus group included several mothers who were battling a chronic illness themselves or were helping to care for family members in similar situations. The most common health conditions that mothers struggled with were diabetes, high blood pressure, and managing their weight. Several were cancer survivors. They mirror many of the health conditions that African American women face nationally.

Overall, the groups were knowledgeable and active about finding health information. They often used the Internet, and scanned magazines and pamphlets for information about a specific health condition. Many of them were also actively involved in the health affairs of friends and family. They routinely gave advice and opinions about what others should do related to health concerns and shared with others their concerns and struggles about their own health. The majority of mothers also actively practiced basic health promotion techniques (i.e., blood pressure screenings, breast exams, regular checkups, etc.), yet their health was often compromised. And, as will be argued in chapter 3, they send mixed health messages to their daughters.

Defining Health

Mothers' definitions about health and what it means to be a healthy woman encompassed answers that ranged from the instrumental—getting regular checkups, scheduling medical tests, and eating certain foods—to an integrated approach. This integrated approach involved receiving social support, creating balance in one's life, and cultivating a spiritual and/or religious foundation. Several mothers across all the focus groups discussed the importance of praying, cultivating spiritual well-being, and having a sense of interconnectedness with other people and the planet as contributing to health. Across all the focus groups, there was universal agreement that health is something that should be nurtured, respected, and that it also is, as one respondent shared, "Essential to whatever dreams, goals you want to accomplish."

In the example below, we see a range of responses that defined how groups talked about health. In the Strategists' discussion, Strategists2 offers a straightforward approach to health, and two other respondents respond that health is about paying attention to what is happening around you and the possible cues your body provides you:

STRATEGISTS2: To me it just means being in a state where you feel good physically, mentally, and keep a check on all those things and paying attention when things don't seem right.

STRATEGISTS3: It's a way of life.

MODERATOR: It's a way of life?

STRATEGISTS3: Yes.

MODERATOR: So what does it mean to be a healthy woman?

STRATEGISTS3: Regular checkups from your doctor, understand your body, how it works.

STRATEGISTS2: Listenin' to your body and not ignoring the signs that it gives you.

STRATEGISTS4: Also listening to that inner voice, sometimes we cut it off when it's, um, trying to tell us that something may not be right or even if you feel well, sometimes I think God gives you that inner voice to let you know, you know, you do need to get checked out or something's not right.

For some mothers, health was considered a "way of life" and an approach to life. Many mothers thought of health more specifically as a state of being that animates and integrates across one's emotions, physicality, and intellect. One participant said, health is "your mind, body, and soul being in sync." Health was reflected in one's environment and helped to order and structure one's life.

In the preceding exchange we also learn from one of the participants that an inner voice may also be connected to a religious belief about God. Many mothers across groups used the language of spirituality, and specifically Christianity, to discuss their understanding of health and wellness and also as part of practices that they use to support their health (e.g., prayer). Nostalgics, in talking about the importance of lifestyle, embody an expansive definition of health, indicating that spirituality and religion can play a role:

> NOSTALGICS1: I agree with others . . . being conscious of what you should do to keep your body healthy is important. So, what you eat and what you do. Often it's moderation. Keeping yourself as stress-free as you can mentally. If you can't control it, just let it go. Pray and keeping my spirit clean and free as I can, which will help everything else because it's all a total package. And then try to do all that and then lead by example.

Nostalgics3 shared that she had several health problems including high cholesterol, high blood pressure, and had polyps removed from her colon and that's why she stays physically active, especially with dance:

> So, that's number one is that I have to do that [stay active]. I'm not as good with the spiritual thing as far as being able to find a ritualistic way of doing things. You know I acknowledge the presence of a higher being. But that whole journey for me has been very difficult. And so I'm trying, again, a process helps me, a process of trying to get better with that. And I've also—I've always been relatively good about focusing on eating well, I try to think about the things that make my body feel better and try to focus on eating those things.

The women go back and forth for several more minutes discussing health and spirituality, some particularly focused on Christianity and a higher power as undergirding the definition of health and others defining it as a sense of wholeness:

> NOSTALGICS1: Health to me is a mind body spirit experience with everything being in line together as a whole person. Your mental health, your physical health, your spiritual health all being positive.

This comment sparks a deepening in the discussion:

NOSTALGICS2: I would go back to also say that, for me, it's [health] not something that's static, like that you've arrived at that point at any time in your life, that it's always, that you're always evaluating and finding new ways for improving your health, whether that's your spiritual health, your mental health, your physical health. And so health is like a process you go through.

Health is not just about the absence of pain. To be healthy takes persistence and recognition of the inevitable ups and downs of life. Maintaining one's health does not always come easily to the majority of the women. Later in the discussion a participant illustrates how she tries to prepare her daughter to manage pain and discomfort:

NOSTALGICS2: I think being able to get from one thing to the next, you know, without [clears throat] too many things falling apart [laughter] makes one healthy . . . If one is able to ride the waves. I remember a couple days ago my child had her first cavity and she had to have it filled. And she doesn't do well with pain. And it was way dramatic, you know. I guess in her mind a big shot of pain. And she was like running around the house and it was like, this is not how we deal with this! [Laughs] And really, like I had to have a discussion with her about how some things are certain in life and one of those things is physical pain. Like, it's going to happen at some point in your life like somewhere and that the extent to which you learn how to manage it and deal with it, the better. To the extent to which you feel you are able to have a healthy experience with things and that there could be ways in which you try to gain control of how you think about it and how you experience it, all of that kind of stuff. That you could even, in your mind, minimize it in some way, . . . you find ways to deal with it.

And I was telling her just like you're at the beach, and the waves and boats are trying to push against her, and that's how you kind of want to think about it. And she seemed to do a little better with it. Not necessarily that it went away or anything like that, but she was not . . . I think the hysteria of it was like making it worse. So, that's kind of, to me, like some day to day like trying my way to manage, you know, what is sometimes the inevitable, you know; disappointment or even the happy things.

The conversation progressed and another person presented their perspective on health as knowing one's limits. This observation is echoed later when we explore the barriers for mothers and the challenges they experienced investing in the self:

NOSTALGICS4: I think a woman gets up in the morning, [just] getting up and keep moving. Keep going even though, again, like your mind is saying you're so tired. But you've got to go out and do what you've got to do on a daily basis.

NOSTALGICS1: And knowing what is healthy for you because it's not the same for everybody. Knowing your limitations, knowing how hard you can push yourself, knowing what to do to get yourself moving, especially with that pain management. 'Cause I feel that way. But trying to be the mother and take the high road and lead by example. Be able to manage certain things and trying to get the daughter to be able to. Like you said, hysteria just makes it worse.

NOSTALGICS2: I think it's a choice, you know. What makes a woman healthy is having access to either the positive, the choice to be positive, to be in control, the knowledge to sustain your body or at least even the knowledge to know what you should do. Even if you don't do it, at least accept the information and some feeling of living in an environment that is safe and comfortable, free of danger and having at least enough sense of control to be able to make the choices. Because I think there's health and then there's existing. And when I think of what makes a woman healthy, I think of choices.

The meaning of health for the groups are about mindset as well as practices (i.e., going to the doctor, eating right, etc.). They are connected to spiritual and religious ideas and to persistence. There is also a tension espoused by several participants, across groups, between assigning responsibility for the individual choices that women can control regarding their health, including "being positive" in one's thoughts and attitudes and negotiating the conditions of the material world either they have faced (e.g., including not having health care, living in a low-resource neighborhood) or have seen others face. Viewing one's health as a choice and more in an individual's control suggests a neoliberal understanding of health. This idea was present across all the groups. That several members in the focus groups expressed this perspective helps us put into context the ways that they see (or don't see) barriers for themselves and their daughters.

Mothering Practices and Inherited Health

The majority of the mothers across the focus groups carry with them strong connections to "folk remedies" and "country" medicine as practiced by their mothers. Many mothers across the groups grew up without consistent health care and have few memories of receiving formal health care except in dire circumstances, either because of the family's lack of economic resources, living in a rural community with a lack of providers close by, or a combination of these two factors and/or being raised by a mother who advocated less reliance on doctors and a more independent lifestyle. Others grew up with mothers who espoused more traditional health-care practices.

These women discussed both the challenges and the opportunities their mothers' health practices had on them. Many cited their mothers as health examples that they were proud of—even if they hadn't had access to formal health care growing up. They also expressed pride about their mothers' ability to do a lot with very few resources and, in some cases, her ability to manage a large household, as some mothers came from a family of seven or more children. Several mothers also noted that they liked seeing their mothers maintain a garden and commented at length about the importance of eating fresh food while growing up, as emphasized by their mothers. For many participants, their mothers stressed limiting the consumption of fast food, either because of access (growing up in a rural environment), or because it was believed to be unhealthy, or both. The most common exercise that people talked about their mothers actively pursuing was walking. The conversation with the Revealers here is representative of how their mothers' health practices were discussed. Moreover, Revealers were also a unique group in that several of the members had living maternal grandmothers:

REVEALERS3: [Turns to another person] My mother's example, I guess, was in many ways like yours. She served healthy food. I used to—I wanted to eat out so badly, but we never ate out. And we didn't have, I mean *never* did have fast food [delivered with emphasis]. And I think part of that was economics. But my mother was a country girl. She always did pick out fresh vegetables. So, I got that from her. And, you know, she didn't exercise, but she worked hard and walked. And she's going on 90 and she's healthy as a horse. And will even chide me about, you know, I'm visiting and I'm eating some cake or pie and she's like "hmm, put that down!" [Laughter] Because she's just, I mean she's serious! You know, she doesn't eat salt. She drinks water. She walks. I mean she eats right. So, I guess I inherited some of that from her. The healthy food, I've started doing that. And even though high blood pressure runs in the family, I think I've adopted a pretty healthy approach as well. I got spirituality from her—the love of God and having that God force in her, believing that.

REVEALERS2: Well, I got my desire [pause], my commitment to exercising from my mother and my grandmother. And my mother is—57, my grandmother is

83. And my grandmother does a lot of walking. But her health stuff sort of ends there. She still smokes. She still drinks, so that's not very healthy.

. . .

But my mother has always encouraged her children, and her two sisters, to be healthy. And then my mother is the, out of the three children, is the one who has the healthiest habits out of the three sisters. And, so I grew up always watching her. She used to walk around her block that we lived on; like if not every day, it was like every other day. I try to do stuff like that. And my grandmother too, I remember my grandmother just recently, like within the past few months when she was visiting the doctor, told me about how her doctor was telling her that whatever she was doing, you know, keep doing it. She said that her doctor told her to always keep her waist trim. And so, you know, that's like her. And I guess she was doing like her version of sit-ups and stuff like that long ago, like when my mother was young and stuff like that.

The Strategists discussed being shaped by their mothers' health choices and we see a mix of experiences. There is the contrast between a woman who goes in-depth about the use of "old remedies" and one that doesn't.

MODERATOR: What kinds of things did your mothers or your grandmothers do to take care of themselves and to take care of you and help you stay healthy?

STRATEGISTS3: They used a lot of old remedies [echoed by others saying yeah, then laughing]. A lot of 'em!

STRATEGISTS5: Well my mama always took me to the doctor, if we had a cough or anything. [others laugh]

STRATEGISTS3: Well, my mama didn't take us to the doctor unless it was severe. It gotta be severe. They used the old remedies, what they grandmothers taught them . . . we did fine by them, so y'all will too.

Moderator asks people to elaborate if she and other participants remember the kinds of remedies used.

STRATEGISTS3: Like when the kid gets, uh, mumps. We didn't go to the hospital for that, chickenpox, we didn't have that lotion, that calamine lotion they put on you now. They had none of that, they put some sardine oil on you [others laugh], there's a lot of different stuff that you know, when we got sick . . . when one kid would get stung by a bee they put tobacco juice on it.

MODERATOR: Did you feel like those remedies worked?

STRATEGISTS3: Yeah, 'cause we didn't know no better, all we wanted to do was get well. So . . . we got well and we didn't go to no hospital . . .

SOMEONE ASKS: Did y'all get better or did y'all just say, "Oh, we feel better."

STRATEGISTS3: No, we got better, and we didn't go to no hospital. And that was another thing, we didn't want to go to the hospital unless we get, um, we cut our hand and it bust open bad and it needed stitches, sometimes even when we needed that we didn't go. She just healed, put things on, wrapped us up and told us to go on and sit down somewhere. We didn't know no better . . . my mother had, there was fourteen of us so . . . she, I guess her grandmother taught her a lot of things, so we didn't go to the hospital for everything.

For many mothers across the focus groups, if they went to a doctor, it was often as a last resort. This was either because of the lack of resources/health insurance, rural isolation, and/or having working parents without a lot of flexibility to leave the workplace. In the exchange above, when one of the mothers is pointedly asked whether she thought the "old remedies" worked, she answers affirmatively. Untraditional health cures were generally discussed in a positive manner.

The Revealers' discussion below also highlights other patterns. The first speaker shared with the group that except for her mother occasionally telling her to reduce salt, there wasn't a lot of health information. The conversation continues with another participant saying that her mother didn't offer much either, just when to wear appropriate clothes so that she wouldn't get ill. And another speaker calls her mother "a nurse" and suggests that she used home remedies, but that she also took her daughter to the doctor:

REVEALERS2: The only thing dealing with health in my family is everybody is hypertensive. So, we grew up with no salt. Even to this day, there is no salt in my home. And that was really the main thing because all through—you can't tell it now—but all through high school I was underweight, way underweight. I was always, you know, my mama was being called in because I didn't weigh enough. I was on vitamins. So, she got called in on a regular basis because I was underweight. But just the salt, dealing with health. It wasn't really discussed. Nothing preventative dealing with health was discussed.

REVEALERS3: I remember my mother kind of being a nurse. I remember just different medical problems from a young age. I remember that I had to wear a cast and this was even before I went to school. I had a cast on my leg because the doctor said I had "water on the knee," whatever that meant. And my mother was always nursing me out of something. I remember having pneumonia and just she would try all these remedies and rub you down all over and wrap you up and make you sweat, and made honey lemon tea. She just did whatever she could instead of always going to the doctor. And that's what I remember. That's why I say my mom is like a nurse. And I'm sure a lot of other people have that experience where, you know, your parent has these little remedies of stuff where they try on you before they take you to a doctor. Not to say that I didn't go to the doctor.

This respondent went on to state that she had unusual leg problems when she was a teenager that required her to go to the doctor often and her mother took her. She ended the narrative with:

> so, through what she did as I grew older, I always knew that on a regular basis I needed to go get a checkup. Or even with my daughter, certain things I'll try before I take her to the doctor. And that rubbed off on me, what she did when I was growing up.

Her comment provides insight into what mothers do differently for themselves and their children. For the mothers that grew up without an extensive formal experience of health care, they utilized that knowledge and sometimes drew on folk remedies, and also took their children to the doctor. They presented themselves as more self-reliant than the mothers that only had formal health-care experiences. They acknowledged that they are already in a different position in that they have health care (unlike some of their mothers), are better educated, and are more aware about health issues. They value having health insurance, but they also value being able to find other ways to care for their children. For other mothers who went to the doctor often, they replicated this behavior, as we see, turning back to the Revealers:

> REVEALERS2: I think my mom was like a stickler for dental appointments or going to the doctor and stuff. And so when I had my children, I took them to the doctor for everything. But now that they're older, I kind of explain why, you know, it's important. Like if I forget and I'm like "OK, it's time for you guys to have a physical." All that is really important to me. And I think that's kind of like what we did about my kids getting physicals every year and making sure they go to the dentist every six months, making sure they get their eyes checked. And to them it kind of seemed like, you know, a little bit much. Like my kids will say "ma, you know, you're doing it too much." I try to remind them this is how my mom was when I was little so that's all I remember, you know. Like we constantly had to go get our teeth checked and we had to go to the doctor for every little thing I guess. I'm thinking that that's the way to prevent something before it happens. Because so many people don't go to the doctor until finally when they go it's like whatever sickness they have is too far gone

or something like that. So, I'm always having the mindset of, OK, if anything's wrong we're gonna catch it before . . . I guess my mom rubbed off on me with her taking us to the doctor so much.

This mother in the Strategists said that her mother did take her to the doctor frequently and she does the same for herself and is also guided by looking at her family's health history:

STRATEGISTS2: I look at my family history and I know I have got to be on top of my game and I try to, you know, tell my daughter that too, I was like you know, 'cause my mother, she died of breast cancer, so I make a point to make sure I do my breast exams . . . I've had a mammogram since I was like thirty years old, 'cause my doctor said, "I know your history so I'd rather start with you now than wait." So I think my family history plays a huge influence on me trying to stay involved in my health care.

There were three inheritance patterns of health practices for participants from their mothers. A third of the participants received little information about health and they had infrequent experiences with traditional medical care. These participants weren't connected to any folk tradition. The second pattern (also expressed for almost a third of participants) was that some mothers were not taken to the doctor frequently, yet still had discussions of health and often experienced the use of untraditional remedies. The last pattern is of mothers who routinely saw doctors and interacted with the medical system and had no experience of a folk medical tradition. Another distinction can be drawn about the mothers' experiences—for several mothers that had no memory of active health care or health discussion, they defaulted to talking openly with their children about health concerns:

NOSTALGICS1: I don't think my mother consciously taught me anything in particular about health. She was a single parent as well. And I just remember her doing everything that she could to make sure that I had everything I needed as well as most of what I wanted. So, I remember her working always more than one job. I don't remember her going out. I don't remember her dating . . . And in my conscious mind, it didn't appear that she was missing anything in her life. It didn't appear that her life was any worse for the wear. But even as I sit here thinking about it, I don't remember her—and I'm sure she dated 'cause I don't know everything she did. But I'm sure she had her party hearty good time nights too [laughter]. But I just don't remember—the most prevalent thing I remember is her working two jobs and always working hard to make sure she could give me everything that, like I said, I needed as well as most of the things I wanted. She cooked healthy meals as far as I knew healthy meals to be back then. 'Cause back then, you know, you didn't run to McDonald's or Burger King. You ate at home. And if you didn't like it, you sure ate it [laughter all around]. So, I remember that. I don't remember going to the doctor for preventative things. I went to the dentist, but when I was in pain and had a tooth that needed to come out. I also don't remember consciously her doing obvious preventative things. So, I don't ever remember us having a conversation about doing healthy things or being healthy. I don't remember her exercising. Of course, back in them days we didn't have health clubs, getting exercising [meant] doing aerobics to a [video] tape.

So, I don't remember any of that consciously, though she may have been doing healthy things that I didn't know about. And she may have been doing things to keep herself healthy. But then, by the same token, she died of colon cancer at 51. And I'm 51. So, the difference that I see, and it wasn't always, is that as a result of that, I have started to look at my physical health differently and to conduct myself in a different way in terms of doing preventative and keeping up with what's going on in my body and trying to be on top of it, and then trying to teach my daughter that as well. I had already created that junk food junkie before, first. So, therefore, I'm trying to go back and undo what I've already done; which is hard.

She elaborates:

But I just keep pointing out to her "this is a known fact. This history is in our family. And it's a direct history because of my mother, your grandmother." I just had my first colonoscopy a few months ago. And I'm saying to her they found polyps, lots of huge polyps, they were of the variety that had we not removed them and I had a colonoscopy when I did, that could have become cancer. And not to scare her, but I said "that's a fact. I'm 51. That's a fact. You need to change your diet now so that when you get my age, you don't have to go through that. You know it's a possibility. You know it's there. Do something about it now rather than waiting until it's too late or waiting to undo something that's already been done.

This narrative moves seamlessly into discussions with this woman's daughter about health and her actions based on her personal history. We pick up this respondent's story along the way and how she began thinking about health as she got older:

I guess I started when my mom died because one thing I said was, when she passed, "I am not going to procrastinate. If something doesn't seem right, doesn't feel right or whatever, I'm going to get it checked then. I'm not going to be afraid to go to the doctor." And pretty much I've stuck to that except when you don't have health insurance. And it's kind of hard to do that when you don't have insurance and when nobody wants to see you for that initial visit 'cause you don't have an insurance card. And you don't want to run up a $2,000 doctor bill since you know you can't pay it or you might spend the next 20 years paying. So, to the best of my ability, I have tried to maintain health insurance.

This participant's story reveals several compelling features that also are present in other groups. In recounting what their mothers did or didn't do related to health practices, often the issue of overwork and the lack of time for oneself marked their mothers' lives. For many, their mothers having had little leisure time and high caretaking responsibilities over a prolonged period may have had deleterious effects on their mothers' health.

Besides Nostalgics1's example of how she acted on her knowledge to support her own health and her daughter's health, there is another important thread to tease out. Her single-parent status is woven throughout her narrative. Eleven of the 24 women were unmarried single parents at the time of the interview. We know that single parents and their children can experience health challenges throughout their life due to stress, financial issues, and lack of support. Others mentioned both their parents' single-parent status and their own, pointing to another part of their inheritance.

Their health inheritances from their mothers have shaped how they understand their own health conditions and communicated with their daughters. And, for some, because of poor experiences or incomplete experiences regarding health, mothers have taken proactive steps to talk with their daughters about their health.

We now turn to exploring the barriers mothers face in maintaining a state of health.

Barriers to Health

All groups identified specific barriers both to their personal health and what prevents women from being healthy in their communities. Diet and exercise were the dominant culprits identified by all groups. Individual women also identified their own challenges regarding barriers to health throughout the interviews. There are also unidentified challenges to their health that were less explicit, but that define their narratives. These challenges are a "low investment in self" and navigating the health-care system.

Only one person out of the entire set of participants stated that they didn't have any current barriers to health. She is a Revealer and talks about having health insurance and cultivating a sense of awareness as a way to keep one's self healthy:

REVEALERS1: I would say I don't have any barriers. I feel like one thing that helps is having good health insurance and planning for those things. For instance, when you have the ability to put into an account at the top of the year that allows you a certain amount of money that is taken out before taxes. And so, you know you have this amount to work with. And so, if you're going to have an exam or whatever may come up, to me I already know something is gonna come up, I'm not gonna be naïve, in a year's time. I know I'm going to have to either get glasses or go to the dentist or need some kind of over-the-counter medicine. And I already know I have a health problem with my back. So, I go to the chiropractor regularly. So, to me, I'm already aware. Awareness, I guess that would be what would be my preventative medicine, is just knowing that I cannot be naïve about my health. It's just a fact of life. You're gonna get sick some time in your life. And just being aware and making provisions for that and making sure you have—like I've worn glasses all my life. So, I know I have to have vision insurance. I know I value having my teeth, so I know I have to have dental insurance [laughter], things like that. I know, like when you get a certain age you have to have these annual exams. So, just being aware and planning for some of those health concerns.

This stands out as a rare comment, the striking exception rather than the rule. Several women mentioned money and lack of insurance as a general concern for women, but not a personal one. As indicated in chapter 1, the majority of the mothers were, except for a few, mostly lower middle class and middle class overall. They had insurance and the ability to take themselves and their children to obtain preventative care. Most did not deal with extreme financial pressures, but instead the grinding challenges of being a working parent and/or a single parent, the realities of multiple caretaking roles with elderly parents, and managing kids with serious health conditions were formidable and mark their narratives.

We Just Give Ourselves Away

Stress often permeated participants' discussion of barriers to health. This was connected both to their work and the intensity of caretaking relationships. In the Revealers' discussion, we see both factors at work. Many of the mothers managed multiple health relationships besides their own:

REVEALERS3: For me, I would say stress at work; the stress of having elderly parents to look after and then maintaining your household. It seems to me, I mean it could definitely affect your health as well as the health of other people depending on how you are, how you're feeling.

REVEALERS5: And for me, my daughter does have a serious health concern and me just monitoring *her takes a lot of time.* Her being the age she is, I ask her if she's taking all of her medications and taking her word and making sure that she is, you know, doing what she's supposed to be doing because, like, just being consistent and staying with her, and just like she [points toward another focus group member] said, other things may pull me away from making sure she's doing what she's supposed to do with her health. [Emphasis added]

What is framed as stress and the juggling of time between themselves and others in their narratives manifests thematically as a health barrier of "low investment in self." With this barrier, as one mother stated cogently, "we just give ourselves away."

This participant in the Nostalgics group highlights what she does to combat the potential for a low investment in self:

NOSTALGICS2: I think it's hard being a parent, and a working parent and putting your needs first to the point where you realize—I think as women we just give ourselves away. And I have to remind myself sometimes that taking time for me is just as important as giving time for my family, my husband, my children, my job. Sometimes I can just *spend myself totally up* and then I remember why I'm so tired [laughs] because I haven't invested in me. So, I think that that is, you know, the choices thing. I mean you can have access to all the trails, the parks, the shoes, the clubs or whatever. But if you don't—that's me. I'll just speak for myself, sometimes just remembering that what's important for my own well-being and health. So, taking that time; that 30 minutes, that 10-minute walk, that—even time in the morning to meditate. I've got to get up at 5:00 a.m. and do something. And when I do that, my day is so much better. I mean I can deal so much better. But if I get up and immediately I'm running and dealing with the kids, then it's like, eh, not good. [Emphasis added]

This mother strives to be proactive in making decisions to mitigate the increasing demands on her time to support herself. In the Experts group, the sense of pressure, tradeoffs between themselves and others, and the challenges of making enough time for themselves were expressed similarly by one of the participants:

EXPERTS1: [T]HINKING that you gotta do so much when you really don't [others agree], thinking I gotta run, I gotta take care of this, oh he don't know what he doin', I gotta go fix that and you're not thinking I probably should stop and go walk around this building or take this pill 'cause it's going to help me later. You're not thinking like that and you're taking care of the kids and oh he's gotta be over here and she's gotta be over here and I don't have two people so I gotta go do it myself. And then you turn around and if you're married you say shoot, he don't know what he's doing [all laugh]. 'Cause that's what it is for me, I'm constantly going and my husband's saying, "Well I can do this," and I'm going, "No you can't, you can't even wash your clothes, I'll do it." I gotta wash the clothes, I gotta do this. You don't think you don't have time to stop and think I need to take care of me. 'cause if I don't take care of me then they really ain't gonna be able to do none of this stuff.

The intensity of the participant's sentiment is evident in the language and repetition of the word "gotta." This sentiment was mirrored in four of the five groups. Another member in the Nostalgics group framed it as the difficulty in creating more time in a day for themselves and having to "steal" it from other places. She talked about the struggle to find "me time" and the difficulty in finding it in the midst of a very busy day.

NOSTALGICS4: My kids always want to sit in the front seat. But, I make them sit in the back. That's my time for myself when I'm putting them in the back. I'm up front, in my own mind. That's, a lot of times, my only "me" time for myself even though they're in my presence. I'm having my "me" time up there. And she [my daughter] talks to me all the way [laughter]. Then I think, "What am I thinking?" especially when I'm thinking, "I know this is my "me" time." That's my biggest challenge, I don't take enough time for myself. I always put my immediate family or my siblings in front . . . It's hard.

This speaker went on to use the words *my* and *me time* emphatically for several more sentences before she finished. Again, the intensity and repetition of the speaker's use of "me" in the comment is striking. She expresses the challenge of locating the self within both a real space (the car) and an imagined space (her mind). This captures both the temporal and spatial nature some women pursue to provide that investment in themselves.

Although Revealers1 spoke most about the importance of individual choices and health, a contradiction emerges in that those choices are unequally structured and that reflects in the unspoken and subtle ways mothers manage their children's health and their health. Naming their frustration with juggling indicated the implicit sense of responsibility of everything resting on their shoulders. Additionally, as discussed earlier, participants expressed the challenges of being a working parent generally and especially being a working and single parent as exacerbating their stress. There was less a language of choice than expectation for most of the mothers. This perception of having to manage and take care of all despite the stresses it places on an individual is a gendered and racialized phenomenon. Black girls and women often experience gendered and racialized socialization that makes it seem normal to take on inordinate and unsustainable responsibilities in the private sphere, especially in heterosexual relationships.

This articulation of low investment in themselves also occurs in the ways that they framed advice to other women; such advice can be viewed as cautionary tales. The mothers, in their roles as friends and co-workers, encourage others (especially other Black women) to make time to take care of health issues, even if they often feel challenged to do so in their own lives. This extended discussion of the Experts is representative:

EXPERTS3: I have a sister and I know she's diabetic. She goes to the doctor when something is wrong, she don't go for a checkup just to, um, make sure I call it, and like they say, I guess it goes back to not trusting. Or always thinking, oh if I go to the doctor they are going find something, I've heard females, especially African American females, say that well if I go to the doctor they're going find something wrong just because of my size or what have you. I have a friend who's really thin, she doesn't like to go to the doctor because she thinks that they're going get on her about being underweight. So, um, I don't know, sometimes it's not wanting to hear what they have to say. Again, that trust issue.

EXPERTS2: I think one of the things I'm always telling my friends and family is don't let it slide like if you don't feel good, and I think women are especially good at thinking, "Oh, it'll be alright, I'll just wait on it." And I've seen that have really bad consequences so I'm always sayin' it's a problem you should probably go get somebody to look at that.

EXPERTS1: It's grown! [All laugh a little, uncomfortable momentary silence]

EXPERTS2: But I think it's something that women especially are like, oh it'll be fine, it's a cough today but it'll be alright, those kinds of things.

MODERATOR: Why do you think that is particularly for women?

EXPERTS3: We're just trying to do too much.

EXPERTS1: Too busy takin' care of everybody else.

EXPERTS3: Yeah.

EXPERTS2: Or other stuff, you know five jobs, four children and you know all those things.

EXPERTS3: And, I think some women don't trust doctors.

EXPERTS1: Or don't understand the urgency of the situation. I know someone that was guilty of going to the doctor and being told this is what's wrong with you, this is what you need to do. And then the person didn't do that . . . and you're just like okay whatever, you know. You don't ever take the medicine, you don't ever do what you're supposed to do, and then you wondering why can't I get up, my head hurts, I don't feel good. You get to that point where you're still not doing what you're supposed to do. You know everything, you have everything in front of you, you just don't do what you are supposed to do to take care of yourself. Oh, I gotta go feed the kids right now, I'll take that pill later, or Oh, I'm just too tired, I ran all day I'm just going to go to bed, I'll take that pill tomorrow.

Diet and Exercise

Across all the focus groups, diet and exercise for both the mothers and their daughters were a source of stress, worthy of constant management and viewed as a barrier to health. Challenges with diet and exercise figure prominently in these narratives. The Nostalgics', Transitioners', and Experts' conversations were dominated by concerns with exercise and diet. They struggled with finding and cooking what they considered healthy food, keeping to a "manageable diet" as framed by doctors, experts, and pundits from TV and the Internet. This was also especially salient for newly diagnosed diabetics in the Revealers, Experts, and Transitioners.

Diet tends to follow exercise as many people talked about both as challenges to maintaining their health. In the Experts' discussion below, notice how the focus on diet returns to the discussion of time and investment of self. The first speaker has just said that her lack of knowledge about not knowing how to "eat right" was a barrier to being healthy and can be a barrier for others:

EXPERTS3: Before I was diagnosed as being diabetic I thought that I was eating right and found out some of the things that I was eating on a regular basis like rice, I had to cut back on, so um, I think lack of knowledge sometimes is a barrier.

EXPERTS4: That's what I was gonna say, you know for whatever reason eating is comforting. I like to read so I come home from work and after doing the stuff I have to do at home I chase everybody away, leave me alone, I'm gonna sit down and read, when I could spend half an hour walking or something, but it's, I guess the perception there's so much stress that I deserve to do what I feel like doing which is sitting around reading a book and eating something. [Everyone laughs in agreement]

In the Transitioners group, the respondent below talked about the challenges of choosing the "right foods" and reading labels, and there was general consensus and agreement about the difficulty. This mirrors other comments across groups:

TRANSITIONERS1: It's sometimes eating the wrong things, not reading labels. I didn't used to read labels at all. You know, I just used to buy things, didn't pay attention to the little small print. And I realized after I got sick and talked to a dietician at work, then I began to read labels because she was telling me the difference in sugars and all that kind of stuff. I didn't used to do that at all. Like now I still do the same—I mean I might eat a bagel. And then I'm on Weight Watchers. So I realize, now, I can't eat a bagel. A bagel is 12 points. And I can't have but 35 points in a day. You don't realize how many points certain things are when you eat them. But it's OK in the morning if that's all you're gonna eat, a bagel and maybe for your snack you're going to have a piece of fruit. So, that's not too many points. But if you want to have more snack things, you can eat like a granola bar and maybe some carrots, something like that or some fruit or apple and not some big bagels. This is what we do, a point system. And so that's what you can do is eat more healthier [sic]. That's my thing. It's working for me.

Later in her discussion about food and its challenges, she added:

And that's the way your body is programmed because that's what your body is used to. Because that's the way, like I said, that's the way I was eating. And in other words, my body is so used to all of these fattening foods, fried chicken and all this starch. I love it. But now I'm trying to do a new thing and change the way I eat so I can lose weight. I *stay hungry* where I used to stay full. I *stay hungry*. I don't like to eat baked and boiled foods but it's best for me. And I've learned to pull the skin off of meat. But at the same time I can eat it. But 30 minutes or an hour later, I'm about to starve again.

The phrase "stay hungry" in this context underscores the amount of focus and commitment it is taking to get to her determined weight on this system. Another person from the Transitioners group adds to the discussion how much she is also trying to work on her health as related to diet:

TRANSITIONERS2: And I said to myself, "You're efficient in your job but you're not that efficient in your health," although I have changed. I don't fry anything. I bake a lot. I bake so much now. I'm up to my eyeballs baking and pasta this and pasta that. So, I said OK, so, you're going to change the way you do—you're going to do more of the things you need to do (about your diet).

Another participant piped up and said diet is the most important thing:

Of course it is, especially for Black women because one, you have, Blacks have a lot of problems with diabetes, high blood pressure, sugar, everything, breast cancer. And it's very important. It is. It is very important to take care of your health.

In discussing the challenges of eating for themselves, the narrative often turns back to meal preparation for the house and specifically their daughter(s). This Nostalgic talks about the intersection between her daughter's eating habits and her own:

NOSTALGICS1: And it's kind of sinking [in]—she's making sort of an effort that she wants to not eat as much beef, not do a cheeseburger every single day, not eat a whole big bag of potato chips every time we have a bag of potato chips, you know, because now I have high cholesterol and borderline high blood pressure—but, I don't feel like I'm sick. I don't feel like I have that kind of stuff. I was healthy as a horse, I thought. I dance like crazy. I exercise. I'm not obese. I probably could eat better. But I know, in the big picture, I know I don't eat the worst I could possibly eat. I'm not a junk food junkie. But I'm one of those that I could go without eating, which is just as bad.

Later on, she adds:

> I cut back on the salt. I cut back on the chips. Cut back on the dadadadada.
> All things in moderation. And if you do it now, then maybe you can save
> yourself from having to do something drastic. [Agreement from others in
> the group]

Universally, the lack of exercise is also perceived as a barrier to their health.
It is a source of frustration, guilt, and sometimes shame. In discussing where
and how they work out, health clubs and gyms are mentioned and some
belong to them, but these are not discussed with enthusiasm. A few have
used personal trainers. Mothers in two different groups mention that they are
in neighborhoods where they don't feel comfortable to walk around at times
when their schedule would allow. Frequent exercise is something that many
of the mothers try to incorporate, as Nostalgics1's comments earlier in the
chapter, about getting up early to squeeze in time for herself, highlight. Like
others during the conversation, Nostalgics2 noted that she was often thwarted
from working out and meeting simple exercise goals due to other planning
and care issues, which circles back to low investment of self.

A similar sentiment is echoed by one of the mothers in the Experts who
discusses her frustration around exercise:

> EXPERTS2: I feel extremely busy. I'm sure somebody else has a busier life than I
> do but I feel like I don't have time for an exercise plan which is something that
> I'm really trying to switch my life around to figure out. But I do crazy stuff like
> park my car way far away from the building and be like okay, if I'm only gonna
> get that much exercise then I'm gonna walk. Okay fine, I'll take the stairs. And
> I work in a building where there is a very large parking lot, so I'll park far away
> and everyone's like, why is your car way down there? 'Cause it's the only exercise
> I'm going to get, you make me sit here in this cube! So those are things that I
> try to do while I try to figure out an exercise plan—just fit in a little bit extra,
> you know walking up and down the stairs, not take the elevator, though it's
> very tempting some days, and just parking far away. That's just how I do it in
> the meantime.

Embedded in their narratives of fitness is the role of support. They often
do not feel actively supported or encouraged by people around them for their
fitness. This respondent has the resources to join a gym and maintain a gym

membership. Yet she identifies lack of support and also feeling conspicuous in a predominately white gym.

> EXPERTS2: I think one of the things that's been a problem for me is like lack of support, like folks around me, I have all these skinny friends who don't exercise, and it's fine for them, they feel like they don't need to exercise, which bums me out, but they're like well, why are you doing x, y, z, why are you paying this money to go stand on this thing. And you know I'm walkin' there, I'm the only woman, sometimes I'm the only woman of color there, so gosh, thanks great. So that's sort of daunting sometimes in the gym, you know, and everybody's so happy to be there and I'm not really happy, I mean I'd rather be asleep than sweating sometimes. I think I lack the support . . . people say you should exercise, but that's not really supportive. I mean it sounds supportive from afar, but it's really not supportive, sometimes it's like preachy. You should exercise. I know! Look at me I know! So I think that's been one of the issues. . . . and my kid is skinny or thin and thinks that she doesn't need to exercise right now and she's very much a girly girl and used to be very into sports when she was younger, played basketball and soccer and now that she's going to high school, she's too cute to exercise. . . . I think that that's one of the barriers for me, well I need some help here, somebody needs to tell me, I don't know, maybe if I knew some other women who needed to walk as much as I did. And I don't, and I just don't have that support in a way that I think really pushes me to do it, so . . . that's a problem for me personally.

Mothers experienced barriers to their health that include diet and exercise. One of the most insidious barriers is the one named stress and juggling of their time, which forms a theme of "low investment in the self." These barriers are connected to the structural inequalities that women experience inside and outside the home.

We might observe that participants have internalized societal neoliberal messages about an individual's responsibility for taking care of their health and can exercise control over their health. While this is an accurate observation, we might also ask, what do they get out of that framing?[1] For these participants I would argue it provides them with a great sense of agency. Many of the participants described the ways that they set about working on certain health conditions. Their focus and commitment to understanding their personal and family histories of health is important. Their commitment to facing their health challenges through an active approach negated or at least provided a counterbalance to their fears about the impact of potentially chronic health conditions. It is possible that at some point this approach will have diminishing returns, but I think it is important to acknowledge the benefits that accrued due to their actions. These benefits included self-advocacy, seeing one's self as worthy of having a healthy future, taking multiple steps to follow health providers' guidelines, undertaking independent research about health conditions, seeing multiple providers, and initiating conversations with their daughters and other family members about health.

Race, Gender, and the Health-Care Experience

Increasingly, health scholars are interested in understanding how implicit racial and gender biases affect the doctor and patient interaction.[2] The women had much to say about their experiences navigating the health-care system and with providers. Much of it was very negative. When it was positive, which was rarer, it was very positive. All groups had at least one person who was highly dissatisfied with their health-care experiences.

Revealers had the highest dissatisfaction with health care generally, followed by the Strategists, who expressed high dissatisfaction, specifically with their doctors. For both groups, this dissatisfaction stemmed from a variety of factors including the inability to schedule appointments, long wait times, experiencing medical errors, and perceptions of incompetence on the part of doctors and staff. For some, cost was an issue. One of the highly dissatisfied women talked about how seeing so many doctors, getting conflicting opinions, was a "turn off" and made her not want to go to the doctor. The prominence of the challenges and expressed frustration across all groups navigating the health-care system and interacting with it forms a hidden barrier for the women in managing and maintaining health. We begin with the Revealers. When the topic of health care arose, Revealer 1 stated flatly, "I'm not satisfied with it." The group became very animated and everyone was engaged. Only one Revealer said she was satisfied with her health care, before this she said, "I'm not satisfied with the cost of it! Another Revealer goes on to talk about the "ineptness of the administrative office" and disagreements she has had with her daughter's doctor, and also that her own doctor hadn't familiarized himself with her files before their visits: "And so it's not always good consistent care. And I think sometimes the administrative side of the doctor's office hinders the medical, you know, side. And that's one thing I'm not satisfied with. But I'm hesitant towards changing to a new doctor."

This conversation continued:

REVEALERS3: I feel like they're always rushing, you know, to move on to the next person; not to fully hear your issues. So, a lot of times I feel like you're just a number and they're all about the money.

In the group, others shared strategies that they used:

REVEALERS5: Well, one way that I try to avoid that, I try to go see the same person all the time, so you can build a rapport with that person. They'll ask me [staff], "well, do you want to see such and such?" And I will say "yes," and I do the same thing with my kids.

REVEALERS4: That may be true but after going to somebody for say over 20 years, they think they know you. So, they think they know this is what you need. And you change as well as them, and sometimes it's not always good to stick with the same person.

Although long wait times and administrative scheduling issues were consistent criticisms across this and other groups, not feeling listened to by medical providers (mostly doctors, but occasionally nurses) also featured prominently in their narratives and contributed to the women's frustration. The Strategists discuss this at issue length. The conversation is first led by one person discussing why they didn't have a good experience at United Wellness and then is joined by another participant who was grappling with a variety of chronic and complex health issues who spoke at length, affirming the first speaker's experience. She then went on to describe her own:

STRAGETISTS2: I've had bad experiences at Conover Hospital with different neurologists, so I just recently just dropped them altogether and went to Dover Valley because I was unhappy. I'd tell them things and try to talk to them, and whatever I said, they'd be like, "Okay, you got 20 minutes, tell me what's wrong." And I'm like well you can't, I mean I can tell you what's wrong, but you can't fix it in that little bit of time, you know what I'm sayin'? So you come in and they're like well I got 20 other patients now you just tell me what's wrong right now.

She tired of this treatment so decided to change doctors:

I made a list for the [new] doctor, he listened to me, he took notes of everything I said, I went in for an appointment at 1:00 and at 1:40 I was out.

. . . And I'm like do you see? When I come to Mercy Hospital my appointment's set for 3:00 and I don't get out 'til 5:00. I'm always the last person out in the doctor's office and I can't understand! I could never understand and I was real frustrated with it, and I was just like, I'm not doin' it anymore, I've had enough so, you know.

This participant elaborated on these points throughout the focus group. She said she would rather travel a longer distance to see a different medical team. Her perceptions were confirmed when a different medical provider admitted that there were errors in her diagnosis. She contrasted her old experience with the new experience with the following: "I like that [it's better] because I want somebody to listen because I'm tired of always having to rush my conversation just to get my point across, you know. And he listened! Even if he didn't care he put on a good act like he cared and he was listening to what I had to say." Self-conscious of what some might have viewed as sharing intense feelings, she ended by saying, "sorry I talk too much."

Other women had very similar experiences and shared her frustration. In this same group, although the speaker below did not identify herself as very dissatisfied with health care, her comments illustrate strategies of dealing with one of the women's complaints—the long wait times:

STRATEGISTS3: Well y'all good if you wait for an hour and see 'em. 'Cause I'm impatient. I go into a doctor's office and I'm like, you tell me one thing, I'm goin' by what you say, if you tell me to wait 15 minutes and you don't see me, I'm in your face in 15 minutes. And so you can come back, and they say, "Oh well it's takin' longer." And I keep goin' back sayin', are you done yet? I mean, once I get in they face and annoy the snap out of them then they pay attention. I say, "I'm not tryin' to be funny, but I'm going by what you say" . . . I'm very impatient and [I'll think] you messed with the wrong one. I'll get frustrated. I'll get up and show my true colors, so I say, "You better just get in there and do what you gotta do." And I'm just point blank, I'm not the one, so let's not start. Sometimes, I'll leave.

The respondent goes on to state that she has strategies and multiple "levels" in dealing with her frustration. She goes in and tries to be nice, and then she gets increasingly annoyed and frustrated, and then when she can't take it, she has to say "goodbye."

MODERATOR: So it seems like you're a little more active with your health care?
STRATEGISTS3: You gotta be, you gotta be 'cause otherwise they take advantage of you. And they'll be like, "Oh, she is just sittin' out there," . . . I'm not doin' it.

This participant described the intense effort that went in to managing herself in the context of medical providers. Interestingly, this respondent, in the

Revealers, who identified no barriers to her health earlier in the conversation, also had similar comments about long wait times:

REVEALERS1: I'm not satisfied (with my health care) because sometimes, number one, the administrative function of the office is inept and I want to ask the doctor what's going on. Why are your appointments always 20, 30, 40 minutes late? Why am I sitting out in the lobby? Why does it take so long for me to get a follow-up? And those things I don't like.

Later in the conversation, she discussed a disagreement with the doctor about diagnosing her daughter. She is agreeing with another participant that said doctors often think they know everything:

My doctor thinks she knows what I need [agreement] and she even puts things on me and my daughter—we see the same doctor—that I'm just not in agreement with. For instance, one time she told me my daughter was depressed. And I said, "My daughter is not depressed." In my mind, like no, she's not. She's just being stubborn. But she took her time and we had like a 30-minute conversation about why she felt my daughter was depressed and that I need to take my daughter to counseling. And I was like "that's not it." And so there are things that I don't like. But I'm kind of, I want to stay with the same person because I want consistent health records. And if something comes up, I'm like, OK, you should be able to go back into my records. But even so, I had something come up recently that I'm thinking, "Why doesn't my doctor know this? This happened before. Why don't they go back into my records and look?"

The challenges with scheduling and long wait times are frustrating. Many women perceived some of the challenges outside of scheduling in terms of interacting as the power that doctors carry in culture. The experience of Strategists3 highlights the level of emotional management that characterized several participants' interaction with the medical system.

As Revealers are having this conversation in describing their frustrations with health- care providers, a spontaneous conversational thread emerged in which they ruminate over doctors and power:

REVEALERS5: Some of us [Black women], we look at them as some type of God or, you know, they've been to school, they're doctors and we're not supposed to question them. And so a lot of times we may get in there and we don't know everything. And you get there and you feel intimidated sometimes. You may have all these questions in your mind you want to ask. But then you forget once you get in there. And so you take this passive role and we kind of just let them dictate to us. But you [addressing another participant] don't seem to be like that [laughs].

REVEALERS1: I found out they don't know! They ask me all the questions. I'm like "Doctor, I'm coming to see you! You're asking me questions. You're supposed to figure it out." Yeah, I question a lot of things. And so I ask for explanations. "Why are you giving me this test, you know? What is the outcome?" But like I was saying earlier, sometimes I just don't get a response fast enough for me.

In order to remedy their dissatisfaction some are quick to choose new doctors, while others feel more stuck. Although not true universally, often women who were raised with the practice of seeing medical doctors had no qualms about switching doctors, while others seemed more reticent. Throughout the groups, there was a unified belief that one would have to be proactive despite the inconvenience of getting to know a new doctor and the transportation challenges of getting to and from multiple doctors' offices.

Doctors

The importance of race and gender of providers to participants was complex. Gender mattered to the women in terms of doctor choice and overall, this preference across groups often trumped race. Most women preferred to have a female provider, and some had been with their primary care doctors for many years. In most cases the female providers for both themselves and their children were white or of South Asian descent. This Transitioner represented common sentiments:

> My doctor is female and she's white. But if I hadn't got Dr. Lafferty, I would have chosen one of the other doctors. She's a Black doctor. I'm trying to think of her name now. I would have went to her too. I like females. I like female doctors, period. It doesn't matter if they're Black or white. I just like female doctors.

Revealers3 is matter of fact about her preference: "That (not having a Black doctor) doesn't bother me because I've never had it. I've always wound up with basically white males. So, you know, I don't really know the difference."

Some women were raised with the idea that having an African American doctor was important to them. And, a few women in the Strategists were concerned about not having a Black doctor, especially as a primary provider.

This preference was in tension as the women frequently characterized Black doctors as mean, harsh, or that they question the doctor's competence:

REVEALERS2: My dentist is African American but our family physician is not. But I'm looking more into that because I'm thinking that just from our own culture and our own kind we know some of the issues that we have. So, lately, the older my kids are getting, I'm thinking we should be going to African American primary doctors just because they know because they probably had the same issues in their family coming up and, you know, they know everything about us.

REVEALERS1: Only one of my doctors is Black—my OB-GYN is Black and the others are all white. But I have no problem with that. I usually try to go—when I first moved here, you know, when you sign up to get a new job, you have to pick your doctors right then and there. And I've been in this area five minutes and I'm picking a doctor. So, I'm like "Okay." But then once I go see them and I've been there, well, I don't want to switch over to somebody else because it's like teaching somebody all over again about you. So, I kind of stay put where I am. But I have gone to a Black dermatologist before for months and months for my daughter's skin. And it wasn't any better (than seeing a white doctor). So, and I was thinking you (the Black doctor) should know about our skin. But, no. I mean what he prescribed was just so way off base.

The Strategists reflected on this issue:

STRATEGISTS3: Well, my kids have African American doctors, I don't.

STRATEGISTS5: Mine too.

STRATEGISTS1: I had one and . . . I think she was kinda mean so she really couldn't help me so I don't know, she was like fillin' in 'cause I went to a place where it was like a group of doctors so you kinda just saw whoever was available. And that one time I saw her I was like mmm, I don't know about her, but other than her I have not had an African American doctor and, it kind of bothers me! [others chime in in agreement]. It really does, I want to see somebody who can really relate to me, you know, on all levels, but I mean . . .

STRATEGISTS5: 'Cause I think us as African Americans, it's different from Caucasians.

STRATEGISTS3: Well, for me back at home I always saw an African American doctor.

STRATEGISTS5: Yeah, well when I was in New Jersey, yes, but I think like where we live it, you know it's just all these Caucasians, so.

STRATEGISTS3: There's a lot of Arabs too, the foreign ones.

STRATEGISTS2: That's what I got.

STRATEGIST55: That's what I got too. I have an Indian doctor too, she's my regular primary care doctor and we see her. My daughter had an incident, with um, she had a boil in her arm, and she had been complaining about it hurting and so we got her in there and it seemed like no one was doing what she was supposed to do and we saw this lady and she took so good care of my daughter. At that point, I was like, I want you as my doctor. And since then we go see her and she knows what's going on. And I like her so . . . I had an Indian doctor and then I had an Asian doctor. I like them, I mean I've never had an African American doctor, I'm sure they're out there but I've never had one.

STRATEGIST54: I had an African American surgeon that I liked, but my husband didn't like, then I had an African American doctor that none of us liked. And I think the reason was because she was not organized. There was like, like you said if you have an appointment at one you might get in here at two and her office was always packed and they were rude, when my daughter was small we were goin' to her and they lost her shot records, I was so upset we changed doctors. So I would hate to say that it was because she was African American, but I mean it was just ugly.

Transitioners were in the middle about their doctors, most preferring to have a Black doctor though some of the members disagreed about the expertise of popular local Black doctors.

Many mothers often expressed a strong desire to work with an African American health provider. However, along with this desire there was a heightened level of frustration with some of the Black providers that they had worked with previously. This contradiction might speak to unconsciously held extremely high standards for Black providers than they would hold for providers of a different cultural background. Another possible explanation is unconscious internalized bias. Minor occurrences within the health-care setting that they experienced with Black providers might be ones that would have gone unnoticed or unremarked upon except for this possible heightened scrutiny. It is also interesting to note that several mothers have maintained Black doctors for their children but not as their own primary providers. This could also speak to the availability of African American medical providers in areas where some of the participants live.

The mothers' perception of how doctors might treat them as Black women was also salient and one where race and gender emerge organically; it reveals concerns about how they will be treated, being the intersection of two communities that are undervalued. The moderator asked a follow-up question to a respondent in the Revealers based on her seeming to say she didn't mind who her doctor was. Prior to this question there was an extended discussion of pain management and the mothers had much to say on that topic. The moderator's follow-up questions sparked this exchange:

REVEALER55: No, listen to me. The white physicians may say that. [Cross-talk] Just because they think that's what we need. That's what we're supposed to do to alleviate our symptoms instead of trying alternative methods first.

    Because if you get this preconceived notion about a certain race, then that's what you think you're supposed to do to get rid of that problem.

REVEALERS3: I could believe that. I mean for them it's just an easy fix and they're going to get—[cross-talk].

REVEALERS4: I agree with you because as soon as you say, "Do you have anything that will quiet the pain?" Oh, that's it!

REVEALERS1: Hysterectomy!

REVEALERS2: Yeah, you do find a lot of women who have had that. Like a lot of my co-workers, that I think are pretty young [agreement] have already had a hysterectomy and stuff before they're even 40. And I'm like "no way!" But if I ran to the doctor, she'd probably say the same thing. Let's do surgery, you know, or [my condition will] become more painful. I may have a cyst or something because then they go away, you know what I'm saying? So, you know, sometimes, like I said, I think African Americans doctors they kind of know because they probably experienced that more so than, you know, white people have.

As the conversation continued, one member spoke up and said that she was very happy about working with her doctor in the present and didn't feel pressured to change doctors.

REVEALERS1: I disagree—well, my experience is different. I think my—my primary care physician is also the doctor I see for OB-GYN issues. And she takes her time. In a way that's good and in a way it's bad because right now I'm going through something. Instead of just quick on it, she'll send me to someone else and get a test. And if she's not satisfied with that result, once they've read something, she sends me to someplace else until she's satisfied with what they saying. [She wants to find out] what is really happening with me. And so, in a sense I'm glad that there's not a quick rush to just send me to treatment because then I would be kind of like "OK, you just found this problem yesterday and the next day you want to send me to surgery?" That would kind of send off a red flag in my mind. So, I'm kind of glad that, even though it costs money, I want to go get this other test because I want to be

100 percent sure that, you know, for instance this problem can't be remedied by any other measure but surgery. I've never had a major surgery and I'm not looking forward to having one. I don't want one! But my experience is different. And my primary care physician is a Caucasian woman. She's probably about 15 years my senior. But she's a patient person and doesn't rush to make a judgment about my health.

REVEALERS5: And a lot of times I think too because you've been with her for so long, she probably understands your personality and your demeanor and you tell her "no," you don't agree with her.

Later, the issue of reproductive health emerges.

REVEALERS3: I'm not happy with the one [doctor]—so I switched. And I mean I ended up having—I went to have a fibroid embolization which was not necessary when I had to go back one year later and have a hysterectomy. And so I just recently switched and went back to a doctor I'd previously gone to. He said, "I wish you had stayed with me and you wouldn't have to go through all that." But just be careful. Just read up and try to make the best decision when it comes to those types of things so you don't have to have two big surgeries.

REVEALERS5: And that's the thing, especially with fibroids for us, our race in general. [Agreement] They are so quick. I mean and that might be the white physician's mindset: "Fibroids, Black women, remove them." But other doctors, maybe African American ones, like you said, will try other remedies to try to, you know, make you better.

Two of the other women in the group stated that they were happy with their gynecologists.

In the Strategists group, one member engaged the group with her perspective about the importance of taking control of one's health:

STRATEGISTS4: I know that you have to take control of it because I was diagnosed with breast cancer in '97 and nobody in my family's ever had it and the first thing I did was I went to the library and checked out like 20 books just because I didn't know that much about it, I mean you hear this and that, but I didn't know what was true and what wasn't and I wanted to be able to sit in the doctor's office and when they say certain things, know what they were talking about. So for me, I had to almost get into a quiet place, inform myself, pray about it, and have a peace within me that what decision I was gonna make was gonna be right for me. Because they will throw a lot of things at you, and you have to make a choice, so um, you know, you have to know what they're talkin' about, what they want to do with your body, and you know, if that's right for you, because there's a lot of things I could've done that I didn't do. I informed myself and I was not gonna be a guinea pig [others agree]. You know because a lot of times they put you in a certain group, just because you are African American or they see certain things happening in the African American woman that they don't see in other women, or they just wanna, you know, they put you in a group where okay, we're gonna see how this thing works on her or, you know, certain groups.

She continued to talk about choosing between several treatment options and trusting her own voice after a lot of reading: "For years we have taken what our grandmothers, our mothers, everybody has told us. And it's not the same. The playing field is not the same. So a lot of times the people that we talk to don't know anything about it either so you know, even, I think [even when] the doctors are good, you trust that doctor and you have good experiences with the doctor, but inform yourself!" This participant affirms the need for women like herself to be active participants in their health care.

Navigating the health-care infrastructure and doctors was a complex process for the majority of mothers. Some participants were satisfied with their doctors and their health treatment. How they would be viewed by providers of both similar and different racial and ethnic backgrounds was salient. Mothers who were able to maintain long-term relationships with their providers were the most satisfied with health care and seemed less worried about discriminatory practices. As the medical community becomes more aware of gender and racial health disparities, it may prompt some providers to interact differently with some of their African American female patients. However, given the concern that many mothers had about their treatment, perhaps some doctors share information in a way that some African American women might interpret as being forward and/or disrespectful or are very quick to make health recommendations based on perceptions of them as a group, instead of their individual needs. Also, it is striking that the Revealers were concerned about reproductive health, given the long and ugly history of Black women's health in this country. Given the intensity of the experiences of both groups and many concerns that participants had about being seen fairly and treated well, ironically navigating the health-care system emerged as a barrier to maintaining their health.

Perceptions of Daughters' Health Risks and the Silence about HIV/AIDS

Mothers across focus groups overall played an active role in their daughters' health. One goal of the original study was originally motivated by a desire to understand the ways that mothers and daughters communicated about HIV/AIDS and what barriers they face in communication and what strategies support communication. When asked the question, what is the biggest health risk facing your daughter that most concerns you, uniformly, mothers did not see STDs or HIV/AIDS as a major concern. No group reached consensus on HIV or other STDs being seen as a number one health risk. They were focused on hereditary or inherited family health issues including various types of cancer, heart disease, and chronic health such as obesity.

Only two people in two different groups—Experts and Transitioners—stated specifically that HIV was an important concern. The Experts discussed HIV (with two people agreeing that it was a top concern) but the conversation quickly returned to a primary concern with their daughters' weight (as it did with many mothers across all groups). Out of the other four groups, one person in the Revealers stated STDs is an issue, one mother raised the issue in the Transitioners but it was not revisited. Instead, as we will see below, the Transitioners were laser focused on the threat of pregnancy.

The importance of being concerned with issues of diabetes and connecting it to family heritage is important; however, equally striking is the silence about HIV and STDs, at a time when North Carolina was a leading state in HIV/AIDS cases, and Black girls and women were and continue to be highly affected. This is partly because mothers do not wish to think of their daughters as sexual beings, and they have a strong narrative of their daughters as virgins. Those frames preclude thinking more broadly about their daughters' sexual interests. Their silence or lack of focus on this issue reveals other concerns and thoughts about sexuality that are discussed here and also taken up more fully in chapter 4.

Weight is the dominant theme that works its way through discussions of health, and this theme intersects with body image and sexuality, and emerges more broadly as a source of tension for the mothers. The Strategists provide a common response for the majority of the groups when contemplating what they see as the biggest health risk facing their daughters:

STRATEGISTS3: Getting diabetes. Because she can inherit, at least my family trait.
And I think, yeah, I think that's a possibility.
STRATEGISTS2: Yeah, my mama had diabetes.

STRATEGISTS3: And breast cancer, and stuff like that.

STRATEGISTS4: Yeah, I would say high blood pressure.

STRATEGISTS3: Yeah, high blood pressure.

STRATEGISTS4: I could run down the list 'cause everybody in my family has it.
   [agreement by several members]

STRATETGISTS4: I tell my family, thank you for this wonderful medical history.
   I thank you so much! [all laugh]

Here the moderator summarizes, "So we've got diabetes, high blood pressure,
cancer, weight, and eczema? Okay." This was a standard response where the
mothers discuss pressing medical issues that are a part of their long-standing
family history. The Nostaglics responded similarly:

NOSTALGICS4: Mine would be hereditary issues. Many family members died
   from them. That was the end of the line for us. Just staying active. At school
   anything that she asks to do—physical activities, I'm game for it.

The participant moved into a lengthy discussion of her daughter's eating habits and her concerns about them. The mothers join in with her and discuss
challenges of getting their girls to eat healthy school lunches.

NOSTALGICS4: Once school starts I don't know if she'll eat much of the school
   lunch. But she's also embarrassed to take lunch, being that she's 12 going on 13
   and to take her lunch is just not cool. That's my biggest thing for this year, a
   challenge for her. A lot of kids eat cafeteria food. I can imagine that it's not that
   good. Well, there's nothing that she really likes that she can take that she won't
   be embarrassed about, you know stuff she can drop in her book bag.

Another mother, Nostalgics2, said her daughter doesn't like much of the
cafeteria food, but will eat fruits and vegetables . . . and that she's generally a healthy eater, but likes to snack late into the night. The conversation
continued:

NOSTALGICS2: My daughter eats relatively healthy when she does eat. But she's
   allergic to so many fruits that make her throat itch, that the only fruit she can
   really eat is apples. And she likes pears and fruit cups with all that syrup and
   sugar. So it's a challenge to get her to eat, or get the vitamins or get what she
   needs that you can get out of fruit out of something else. She's pretty OK with
   the vegetables . . . so I'm not worried about that. It's funny you were talking
   about her taking lunch 'cause my daughter loves Chinese food; which I like

OK, but the Chinese restaurant that she likes to go to and get it, to me, is greasy and just ugh! But she likes to go there and she gets chicken and chicken lo mein. And she gets that because she knows she can eat some that night and then she can take some the next day. Now, I'm a gadget person even though I'm no "Susie Homemaker," but I have every gadget that you can— and I have all these cutesy containers and blah, blah, blah. She will take it to school in that Styrofoam container. [Laughter] And I'm like, "Is that not 'country'? You mean you're actually going to take that to school? I've got all these containers in here. Why don't you put the chicken in there?" "No, no." So, I'm aware of the embarrassment part. She's not embarrassed to take that piece of Styrofoam with her. [Laughter] But I guess the biggest issue is just getting her to eat healthy because, like I said, I created this junk food junkie. She'd rather eat out than to eat a home-cooked meal any day.

I don't have to worry about her being physical. She does eat late at night. But she's like me. When I was her age, I was real thin and ate all the time. And it didn't affect me. Of course as you get older—I'm still not that huge but, you know, I still feel it. And I tell her just keep it [weight] down. Look at your daddy's mama and look at the older folk in my family and you know that's where the potential is. So, you can eat what you want to now, but just keep that in mind.

The conversation continued as they pursued talking about their daughters' food preferences and school lunches:

NOSTALGICS2: I'm interested you mentioned snacks and school lunch because my daughter did reach a point where she wouldn't take lunch. So, we started giving her lunch money. And then I realized she wasn't buying lunch. So I asked her, "What are you eating? What's for lunch?" And she was having cookies and she said, "I hate their lunch." And then I realized she's not really buying food. So, I started making her eat breakfast. It's like I can control breakfast and dinner. But I can't control lunch. I just gave up on lunch because I'm convinced she's not really eating lunch. She's buying cookies and snacks. I mean I don't know. So, my concern is just she doesn't eat enough vegetables and also doesn't get enough sleep.

This pattern is repeated across the focus groups. The main focus that arises during discussion about perception of risk to daughters' health is on healthy eating and minimizing excessive weight gain.

In the Revealers they also talk about food and weight as it arises in connection to a specific health issue for one of their daughters:

REVEALERS3: Obesity.

REVEALERS2: Mine would be obesity and probably diabetes.

REVEALERS4: I would say breast cancer and diabetes because it does run in our family.

REVEALERS5: I'm concerned with my daughter. She has always been overweight and we didn't know why. And two years ago we found out that she had a disease that was causing her to be overweight. She had Acanthosis. She had a lot of hair on her face. And we've had to go to a sugar-free diet in the house, which is good for everybody. At first it was hard to get the other kids on that bandwagon.

REVEALERS2: Right, right.

REVEALERS5: It's either water or diet drinks! So, it's been a lot these past two years. So, the same thing, the obesity. But, you know, we might not like to talk about it but the first thing that pops into my head is, oh, she's 15. She's in high school. And we like to think that we teach our daughters to abstain from sex and everything. But I think about STDs and if something is going to happen, please God, watch over her. We preach abstinence. But I'm not so crazy and naïve to think that that might not happen. So, STDs, definitely.

It's hard to know if this respondent was talking about a particular STD or HIV/AIDS. Interesting to note that no one ever returns to this as a part of the conversation.

Let's look more closely at the two groups in which STDs is mentioned as some of the mothers' number one concern. A closer examination reveals that HIV is mentioned and it is within one of the two mothers' groups who may be more inclined to talk about sexuality because among them are a medical doctor and two health educators. In the Experts group, one person clearly says HIV outright out and another person agrees. Notice, however, how weight comes back to being the issue:

EXPERTS4: AIDS.

EXPERTS1: Yeah.

EXPERTS2: That's the big one, I mean, like the preventable things I think she can get that, and AIDS is preventable but I think she doesn't see it, I think it comes to her like yeah, those people. And I actually have done a lot of health education about STDs so I've shown her pictures of a herpes lesion, I've described gonorrhea, like I can do all those things but for her it's like oh that's, I just feel like the numbers are so bad that she's walking in a mine field. I mean I know that seems sort of harsh but that's the way I see it, it's a mine field out there and I'm just trying to help her navigate and it's so difficult when people are like oh it's not a big deal and blah blah blah and whatever, and like I know the numbers,

I've crunched the numbers, and they're not good numbers! Like it's scary like there are a lot of mines and you know, I just, that's my big fear . . . but I also might be slightly paranoid!

EXPERTS3: I think gaining weight, because she'll run track and I kind of forced her to do that because I felt like she needed to do something, she does nothing. I felt like she needed some other extracurricular activity. So I told her she had to make a choice, she had to do something, some people said I shouldn't have forced her but now she likes track, she wants to run again. She dances, she likes dance, I just try to stress with her the more she's active the less likely she will gain weight and get, because I feel like gaining weight or being overweight is a lot of um, or leads to a lot of diseases and I'm speaking from personal experience because I've also been told that I have sleep apnea which is weight related. I know I might not be like a lot, but when you're used to being maybe a size seven, eight, and then now a size, I don't know, eighteen, it was an adjustment for me and I'm finding out you know sleep apnea, maybe later on heart disease. My grandmother has it, my mom has high blood pressure and asthma, all these things you know, so my thing to her is just watch her weight. I know it's hard, but I feel like with lifestyle changes it can be done. Just because she's all thin now doesn't mean she'll stay that way so she's got to work on it and don't take it for granted because I think I did that too. So . . .

EXPERTS4: I have four kids and three of them are very slim and one of them is normal to plump and he had a really hard time with that and then and it made talking about exercise and food at our house very difficult because the ones who were slim had no concerns, nothing to worry about, didn't have to do anything and so . . . My daughters clearly need to exercise, they both happen to be thin but they need to exercise and they don't. I don't know how to get that across, that's a good thing [to exercise] that makes you feel good, especially my younger one who has a tendency to be sort of melancholy and sort of a hypochondriac and if she would just get out and do something I know she would feel better.

They get more engaged in this discussion:

EXPERTS3: But I don't want her getting to trying to stay thin and being unhealthy and getting anorexic or bulimic, and that's one of my concerns for her 'cause she's so confident, but she's so concerned about how she looks and it's scary because I feel like because sometimes she won't, she'll say she's full. She'll say, "Oh, I just ate something at home I'm not hungry." What did you eat three hours ago? She'll say, "Nothing, or maybe a bowl of cereal or something." [to the group] It's like y'all don't know I eat, I eat! Then see, my family are well, my mom's overweight, my grandmother was, so she's looking at all that, then her dad is telling her better watch out or you're going to end up like your mom. And I'm like don't do that, because she's 13 and she's so vulnerable right now and I'm just scared that she'll hurt herself trying to stay thin the wrong way, because I know that it happens. A lot of people don't think that it happens to African American girls but it do.

EXPERTS4: Sure it does.

EXPERTS3: I had a friend who was anorexic and she was almost kicked out of college because of it. It was a health risk at the school. So that is one of my biggest concerns with her.

Later in the conversation Experts2—who agreed that HIV/AIDS was a concern—discussed how she worries about scheduling her daughter's time and that she is also taking her to HIV seminars that her church holds, after describing herself as "nosey":

In our church, they do a lot of HIV/AIDS seminars and I make her go and she's like "Oh I don't want to go again." Yeah, come on, because you need to know this stuff, find out what's going on, find out what's going on in the community. We go out and work in the community with a lot of HIV-positive people. So, one, she's not fearful of someone, but by the same token she'll understand this disease and what it can do to somebody. And then she won't be so gung ho to go out there and just settle for just anything. Because it could have been, it didn't necessarily have to be sex that brought that disease, but it could have been a drug needle, it could have been a transfusion, it could have been anything.

It is interesting to note that, although HIV gets discussed, overall the conversation is mainly dominated by concerns about their daughters' weight and other health issues. Experts2 agrees with Experts4 about the importance of HIV, but then they never discuss it further. Experts2's discussion yields that she has taken action on how to discuss HIV issues with her daughter.

The Transitioners wrestled with the question and it elicited a more direct discussion of their fears and concerns about sexuality than any other mothers' group. They needed the question repeated and they struggled to reach a consensus. They begin by discussing peer pressure and how they believe boys are motivated to do and say anything to have sex with their daughters:

TRANSITIONERS1: Peer pressure and all that stuff I imagine that they want to try and do.

TRANSITIONERS2: The boys.

TRANSITIONERS3: Little boys saying the same thing they were saying back in the day. [Agreement] [Cross-talk]

TRANSITIONERS4: They tell you all that sweet nothings in your ear. And, they do that to get in your pants. [Agreement]

TRANSITIONERS2: My focus wasn't even on boys at the age of 13, hers is. And that's where I have a problem.

MODERATOR: So, that concerns you for her health?

TRANSITIONERS2: For her health, it concerns me—peer pressure. We've talked about birth control. "Well, I'm not at that point yet, grandmamma." Well, you know, my opinion is you're going to get to that point, you know what I mean? "Well, I'm not ready." We had an argument in the doctor's office about it because Kenya's period started. It's bad enough she's a 34DD bra and she's not but 15. And I said to her, "I want to put you on some type of birth control." I said, "It's not saying that I'm giving you permission to have sex. I'm just saying this is for your protection because I know things happen." I'm not crazy. I was a teenager one time. I can't be everywhere. And that was mostly what I was concerned about. But she said, "Well, grandmama, I haven't done anything yet." I said "OK," [Then] I sat down and told her. I'm very open. I've been very open with my children. They can always sit down and talk to me about anything. If I'm not sure, I go down to the health department and get pamphlets or I go get a book to read up on it. But that's mostly what I was trying to talk to her about, and that mostly about her health, you know. That was my thing.

Transitioners2 engages in a long discussion about the challenges that may arise for her granddaughter, and she worries about possible sexual relations.

TRANSITIONERS2: It's all of it. [Cross-talk] All of it concerns me about her health. It's all of it.

TRANSITIONERS4: You can tell if they're sexual.

TRANSITIONERS3: That's true.

TRANSITIONERS2: You know, that's why I try to teach my kids. [repeats her concern about boys whispering sweet nothings in a girl's ear] And you started your menstruation and you're like "OK, my mama ain't gonna know it." [Agreement] And then you turn around and you do have sex. [Cross-talk] Condoms. You can talk about condoms. They can talk them out of a condom [agreement]. And then AIDS lies everywhere.

ANOTHER RESPONDENT: That's true.

TRANSITIONERS2: Then if that happens, it's over, your life is over, you know. [all delivered emphatically] Because we're talking about something you can never,

ever get rid of [agreement]. I mean the only way out of that, is death. So, that is, to me, a very big concern when it comes to kids' health, adult's health, anyone.

At this point in the conversation, another speaker says someone she knew was misdiagnosed with HIV. Transitioners1 jumped in and emphasized how doctors can get diagnoses wrong, and that it is important to rely on a higher power—God:

TRANSITIONERS1: Let me tell you like I tell it. I will tell anybody. Doctors actually only have the knowledge that God gave them. They don't know everything. [Agreement] And sometimes—and I'm gonna tell you what, I have seen it happen, a lot of times a doctor, doctors can make mistakes just as well as we make mistakes.
TRANSITIONERS5: That's true.

One of the participants stopped the flow of the story, which was being dominated by Transitioners2 and the idea of doctors misdiagnosing HIV, and said, "Read that question again." The moderator read the question and she definitively answered, "Getting pregnant too early." There was discussion and then group agreement. The moderator acknowledged the consensus and moved on. Additionally, Transitioners2 went on to talk more about challenges with sex than HIV/AIDS per se.

In the Transitioners group, HIV functioned both as something openly named, unlike in other groups, and was also alluded to as death. As we will see later in chapter 4, HIV and STDs are on the minds of the mothers—worry, yes, but not always in a way that necessarily led to action or potentially to discussion. They see it as a sex issue, but not always as a health issue.

As other scholars have noted, attention over the last two decades has been placed on childhood obesity in public health campaigns. Mothers' dominant concerns were managing their daughters to maintain a healthy weight and what to do about school lunches. Perhaps this should not come as a surprise, given the past 20 years of waves of public health announcements that emphasize the threat of obesity. The "fat body" as one that needs to be managed through food, dress, and sexuality is relevant here. Kids of color (explicitly or through media representation in news stories) have been a dominant focal point for the media and experts. The mothers' concerns may mirror some of their own concerns about healthy diets, the politicization of food choices, and mothering, and serve as an extension of their maternal control. Regardless, this focus leaves little room for thinking about HIV.

These concerns have ongoing implications for public health approaches. The fear of HIV does not seem to have a strong hold on the mothers. They are more concerned with teen pregnancy and general sexuality. This suggests that public health interventions may need to develop new and creative strategies to encourage a renewed focus on risks of HIV that consider how race and gender structure parental narratives about power and pleasure for young people, especially girls of color.

Conclusion

These women spend time thinking about their health, talking to others, and making sense of their health conditions. There are many ways they work to keep themselves healthy. Some of the women struggle with some of the same structural challenges as their mothers, caretaking and long working hours that leave little time for dealing with stress. The mothers have internalized gendered messages that implicitly construct the mother as the person primarily responsible for all caretaking related to health and the consumption of healthy foods. This internalization leaves little room for questions about the way fast and cheap food is easily obtainable in their communities. The invisibility of the well-organized lobbying efforts of companies that manufacture processed foods and companies that serve meals in public schools is also obscured.

The women as a group also have better health care access than their mothers did and are trying to make informed choices about their health. They see their doctors regularly and get checkups. But the challenges that face them deal with working within a medical system that is highly bureaucratic. Many of them mentioned being dissatisfied with various medical providers and searching for better options. Some were highly attuned to how being Black women can negatively impact how doctors treat them and what kinds of treatments they will be offered. This raises the question about the ways in which doctors understand issues of health disparities and how they see their patients. I argue that given negative experiences with medical providers by many participants, interaction with the health-care system constitutes an external barrier. One of the major risk factors for their daughters' health was under the radar. Now we turn to how the daughters both view their own health and understand their mothers' health.

3

"I'm in Between"

Daughters and Health Inheritances

How do young African American girls, in this study, discuss their health? What does health mean to them? What stories do they tell about their mothers and grandmothers? Do they perceive any barriers to their health? If so, what are they? What has been their experience with medical providers? Rarely is there an opportunity to delve deeply into how young African American girls perceive their health and the health care that they receive. This chapter explores perceptions of their health and their mothers' health, their barriers to health, and experiences with medical providers. It explores the nature of communication about their health between them and their mothers.

Daughters have many inheritances that shape their experience of health. As we gleaned from chapter 2, many mothers have tried to model healthy behaviors for them that relate to exercise, choosing sustaining foods, and a positive mindset. Like their mothers, they inherit a folk tradition that stems back to their grandmothers, family members that they highly value. Several of the daughters have close relationships with grandmothers and gave examples of receiving health advice from them. They also as a group have had access to health care when it was needed. The other face of those inheritances is that some daughters are raised in families that are single-parented, and many have parents that work two jobs. This means that mothers are under various types of pressures and may have a difficult time both prioritizing their health and attending to their daughters' health. Many also live with mothers who struggle with a variety of chronic and sometimes debilitating health issues and who may exhibit contradictory behavior when it comes to diet and exercise. As we will see in this chapter, the messages daughters receive around health sculpt their ideas about sexuality. These inheritances are creating ripples of meaning in the daughters' outlook and attitudes about health and well-being.

They knew basic information about how to stay healthy, including where to find health information. Yet they often did not think of themselves as healthy and they struggled daily with their choices around diet and exercise. The majority of girls in only one of the five groups (the Romantics) answered a definite yes to the question, "Do you consider yourself healthy?" Overall, the girls could and did describe the general context of health. It is in the ways that they describe themselves as unhealthy that provide insight into their own struggles and how that mirrors their mother's challenges. Girls also have mixed feelings about health-care professionals, with few having positive responses.

Two groups throughout this chapter tend to stand out as dynamic opposites: Romantics and Loners. The Romantics as discussed in chapter 1 tended toward an optimistic, positive, and friendly worldview. The Loners, in contrast, tended to present a worldview that expressed frustration, independence, individual reliance, and disconnection. The Romantics were the only group in which *all* members described themselves as healthy. They also had the most sophisticated and broad-ranging discussion of health. Additionally, they tended to describe their mothers as healthy. The Loners stood out among all the focus groups, as all the participants categorically described themselves as not healthy. In addition, most of the Loners did not describe their mothers as healthy. We begin with their definitions and perceptions of health.

Defining Health

Across all the focus groups, girls were able to name several main components of health. When asked about what makes a woman healthy, the majority gave responses that described health as a set of tasks and common behaviors that included: eating right, eating vegetables, avoiding junk food and oily and heavy foods, drinking a lot of water, and not smoking. They also noted that possessing certain attributes (e.g., having pink gums and bright teeth, which may indicate being a nonsmoker) typically indicated health. The ability to stay healthy was also linked to being a consumer. Staying healthy, for a few girls, was about maintaining one's outward appearance, and this dovetailed with a type of gender performance, including buying clothes, perfume, and female-oriented products.

There were a few girls across the groups that answered "I don't know" (what health means), or said because they were not yet a woman, they could not comment on what it means to be healthy.

Mindset

The girls described health through a mindset lens connoting both what one thinks about one's self as well as "how you present yourself in the world." Many stressed the mental image of what you think about yourself as connected to health. A participant in the Romantics summarizes another girl's comment for the moderator: "She's saying it's about your self-esteem, how you feel about yourself, how comfortable you are with your life." This mind-set approach involved confidence and self esteem, and girls said that being healthy means feeling good about themselves, their choices and, notably, their bodies:

> I think health means that I feel happy about myself and I'm satisfied about my-self and the things that I do that I'm satisfied by my life. I don't really think that it's about how skinny I am or that kind of stuff. 'Cause I may be skinny, I may have a real good life but I just may not be happy. Because I'm physically healthy and emotionally healthy, I feel good about myself.

For some girls, mindset was also expressed through behaviors, especially gendered ones:

> It's your whole demeanor, like your presence. It's, like it depends. Like, OK, if I just came in here and I sat like this or whatever, you know, that really wouldn't be, well, that's not lady-like. So, if you came and crossed your legs, you know, speak with intelligence, you have good posture, you know.

Cleanliness

Cleanliness was a consistent descriptor across all the groups as a char-acteristic of health. All of the focus groups stressed cleanliness as being connected to health and being healthy. Being clean was a prominent factor across the focus groups, both in the girls' own estimations and when asked about what their mothers told them about health: "Keep yourself clean" was a phrase that daughters said they heard a lot from their mothers. "Musty" was a popular term in many focus groups. To participants, musty meant having a strong body odor. As this respondent shared: "If I walk around musty or something, she [her mother] will like call me out on it in public. She'll be like 'Raise your arm.' and she'll be like 'MmMm . . . No!' Like she will call me out." Cleanliness was not just a physical trait but was also used to indicate a state of spiritual health. For some of the girls, like some of the mothers, health indicated a relationship between emotions, the physical body, and also what some girls referred to as "the soul," or essence. They often used the language of Christianity. In two focus groups, girls emphasized the importance of "being clean with God." The daughters discussed the concept of repenting for one's sins and doing what is right in the eyes of God. One daughter stated that her mother taught her that you should think about what Jesus would do in a similar situation before you act (thereby using Jesus' behavior as a standard or benchmark from which you should model your own behavior).

Responsibility

Being healthy is also intricately tied to being responsible, as was mentioned across four groups. Responsibility means several things: being relied on and trusted, taking on more responsibility for one's self and in one's environment, and how individuals handle themselves in difficult situations. In this exchange in the Romantics, a young woman works out her criteria and meaning of health:

Yes. My body's healthy and my self-esteem, how you feel about yourself, is strong.

I would say yes I'm healthy, but no one's gonna be perfectly healthy. Like I'm not perfectly healthy. And like some say that I'm too skinny for my age. I'm not. I'm just small. But I do, I eat right, I exercise right, so in my mind I'm healthy.

. . .

[Sometimes] I'm not as comfortable with myself as I should. And I don't show it 'cause, like, a lot of my friends, they'll have problems and stuff. And I'm always, like, the strongest one out of the group. But I don't never show my problems—I don't ever show that I'm not all, like, I love myself, this kind of thing, like I tell them they should be. So, right now, no. But I don't know, I think—I'm going to start working on that because I can't be telling people to love themselves and I don't always love myself. That just don't make no sense.

As stated before, the Romantics tended to have a more optimistic and sophisticated perspective about health in comparison to the other groups. However, one does wonder how the idea of responsibility and strength also play into this respondent's understanding of being healthy and how this will influence her later. The internalization of "the strong Black woman" trope and its effect on African American women is an ongoing area of scholarly inquiry in political science, in public health, in sociology, yet few have searched for its possible origins in Black girls' developmental experiences.[1] I was struck by how many girls used the language of responsibility in their definition of health. This might suggest that they believe that they can or should control situations that are beyond their immediate sphere of influence.

Conversations with Mothers about Health

When asked what their moms told them about staying healthy and what conversations they had with their mothers about health, the daughters most often divulged thoughts about sex, relationships, and food. Food and weight play a central role in discussions of what they can recall mothers telling them about being healthy. The girls disclose mothers' transgressions with food. They also praise mothers for their vigilance with reading nutrition labels and food preparation, trying new foods, and cooking with low-fat ingredients. Their narratives about what their moms tell them about health reveal insight into what gets privileged and retained for them, and also echoes some of the struggles that the mothers experience, as discussed in chapter 2.

Most of the girls, when asked, "What does your mother share with you about staying healthy?" answered in an "everybody knows this" tone without much emphasis. As if this information is indeed what *everyone knows* (and perhaps they cannot believe we are asking them these questions), they respond: Eat right, do not eat junk food, and exercise. For example, in the Distrusters group, one girl offered, "I can't eat a lot of salt. I can't eat a lot of junk food. And I have to take care of my hair and my clothes, everything." For many, the discussion throughout the focus groups deepens as the conversation evolves, and it often turns to food, sex, and relationships. They add that their mothers have also told them, "don't have sex, don't use drugs, and learn what it means to be in a healthy relationship."

In the Equalizers, a participant (Equalizers1), recalled a conversation with her mother about weight: "She told me that I eat too much and I went to the doctor and . . . gained too much weight. So me and my mom had a conversation about eating healthy, but it didn't work." The participant indicated that there were no follow-up conversations after that.

In the Romantics, after debating the number of glasses of water one is to drink daily and one girl saying that her mother told her to "not eat a whole lot of junk food," the conversation turns to her mother's behavior. She immediately follows up with, "My mom says that but she'll buy me ice cream sometimes!" [Laughter from the girls] This comment speaks to the implied contradiction in several of the focus groups between what mothers say and what they actually do. Beneath the playful surface these comments can indicate how daughters notice and sometimes judge mothers about their inconsistencies, as we will see in the next section.

In many of the groups, conversations about sex and health overlapped prior to any questions about sexuality, which means that in some of the girls' minds, health and sex were overlapping ideas. After saying that she could not remember anything specific about health, this participant in the Romantics talked about what her mother had shared with her about relationships:

ROMANTICS1: She's like, do not get in a bad relationship.

MODERATOR: So, what's a bad relationship?

ROMANTICS1: Getting in one. In the first place, if you need to ask then you're in trouble.

ROMANTICS2: Thank you.

ROMANTICS1: Someone that might hit you.

ROMANTICS2: Someone who's disrespectful.

MODERATOR: So, what would be disrespectful that a person would do?

ROMANTICS3: Like they come to your door and they ask for you and then your mama come on down and they might say something to them like that's disrespectful that's not nice.

[Someone starts talking]

MODERATOR: [turns] You were saying?

ROMANTICS3: My aunt always says if you have a boyfriend and he talks back to his family and friends and others, then he's not a good husband.

MODERATOR: What's a good relationship? What's a healthy relationship?

ROMANTICS3: I mean he likes you and he'll be like, I mean he don't call you names. Like, he's not rude, he's gonna be nice to you every morning instead of saying things that . . .

ROMANTICS1: I think a good relationship is when, like, you're comfortable with a husband and you enjoy being around him.

ROMANTICS4: I believe what she [points to another participant] said, that you are comfortable with that person and you like being around them and they make you feel happy.

ROMANTICS2: A person that don't like you for your physical appearance, but what's in your heart.

The conversation around relationships branched into discussion about sex, and other girls jump in to answer the original question:

ROMANTICS1: We talk about different things. Well, every once in a while me and my mom get to sit down and we talk about girl stuff.

MODERATOR: Give me an example, like, of girl stuff.

ROMANTICS1: Boys. Usually I can talk to her about a lot of stuff and she understands but [inaudible]. We talk a lot. And there can be rules.

The conversation continued and then, like in the Distrusters group, the Romantics identified grandmothers as people they talk to about health and other matters of importance. Talking to someone was an important part of staying healthy for these girls. They were better able to recall what kinds of things constituted taking care of their health than specific conversations with adults. This finding is in tension with many of the mother groups that expressed they regularly talked with their daughters about health.

Barriers

Diet and Exercise

The sense for many daughters of being "in between" as they describe their state of health and having to navigate health is striking. Given the prominent position of diet and exercise in the girls' narratives, these constitute barriers to health. Barriers to health from focus group comments mirror challenges that were identified by the mothers in chapter 2. As reflected in the mothers' narratives, when the daughters do not describe themselves as healthy, food and exercise are the common determinants. Black girls also commonly face structural barriers to health that include disproportionately living in neighborhoods that are economically under-resourced and that have higher rates of violence, especially sexual violence, and educational inequalities.

When girls perceived themselves as "not healthy," they most often talked about diet and exercise. Their answers emerged organically without them being directly asked about barriers. The way they discussed their health often shifted when talking about food and exercise, and they often employed self-denigrating talk. This is where blame and shame arose and became pronounced. They repeatedly used the words, "laziness," "lack of self-control," or the phrase, "I can't help myself" in describing their failure to be healthy.

Besides diet and exercise, other barriers that impact health for some of the daughters that emerge from the focus groups are balancing working and parenting and minimizing their exposure to smoking. Their emphasis was on diet and exercise, showing a tendency to focus on their own behavior rather than environmental or structural factors.

The next three examples point to the moments of shift that trigger negative evaluation of their health related to diet and exercise. We begin with the Equalizers.

MODERATOR: So would you describe yourself as healthy? No? [Girls laughing quietly; almost all say no]

EQUALIZERS1: A little.

MODERATOR: Why or why not?

EQUALIZERS1: Because I don't eat healthy. [Everyone laughs]

MODERATOR: So a lot of it has to do with the diet?

EQUALIZERS1: And, I don't exercise.

EQUALIZERS2: I exercise, but don't eat healthy at all! [Delivered with emphasis]

MODERATOR: Okay.

EQUALIZERS3: I exercise, but I don't eat healthy either.

MODERATOR: A lot of you are saying that you don't eat healthy. What does that mean? How would you define a healthy diet versus a diet that's not as healthy, as you're saying?

EQUALIZERS3: I eat a lot of fat. [Skeptical looks from other girls] I'm serious, I do. And I eat a lot of times a day. I don't know why, but I eat a lot, just being bored I just eat.

EQUALIZERS2: Me too. I woke up yesterday and I ate like a bag of chips and some candy bars, and then I went and like walked around the block, or ran, I can't remember what I did, and then I came back and quickly ate more stuff. So, not exactly a healthy diet.

A few things are worth noting in this exchange. First, girls were able to identify the types of food that are considered unhealthy, and there was widespread agreement. Across the focus groups there is no mention or embrace of the action of dieting (i.e., going on a diet, planning a diet, facing challenges of being on a diet, etc.) as a way to talk about managing their weight. Diet referred to foods that they consumed, not a program or regime. Often girls said they exercised to "be in shape," but did not mention counting calories or caloric restriction. Although this kind of exchange is seen as normal in many girls' lives, particularly of a specific class and racial/ethnic background, there was no evidence of that here. Many scholarly discussions of girls' eating behaviors have focused on the degree to which excessive dieting and other "disordered eating" is present. In this exchange there is an initial lightheartedness to the discussion, but that should not minimize the importance and relevance of the girls' often negative self-perception. The typical way of framing weight challenges isn't evident here, but that doesn't mean some of the girls don't experience any struggles with their perception of weight.

This next example from the Moderates also highlights the speaker's self-accusatory shift when food is discussed:

MODERATES1: Because I'm like always on the go, because I work now and I'm always going to and from work and so sometimes you go to McDonald's and stuff like that. So in food ways, I'm not healthy.

MODERATES2: Yeah, me too.

RM: Yeah, me and food we get along well, we get along very well.

MODERATES3: And, I know what effect that has that's not always the best, but you know I try to eat healthy. I try. My aunt's been down here so she's been doing the whole vegetarian thing.

[Cross-talk about eating vegetarian]

MODERATES4: Like, I have a couple of salads, every once and awhile. I'll eat a decent meal and I'll try to have like all my healthy foods put into it.

For mothers, challenges around maintaining a healthy diet revolve around their caretaking roles, employment, and stress. In contrast, several daughters talk about boredom and laziness as a main explanation for their behavior. One respondent in the Equalizers stated that her mother tries to keep her from "doing unhealthy things, like watching too much TV and stuff like that, like being in the house being bored, having nothing to do." She noted that she is often bored. The conversation continues:

EQUALIZERS1: I make the choice. Like, I think her, my mom tells me to eat healthy, she buys grapes and things and tries to make me eat. And I'll eat it but I mean, I think I make decisions not to be healthy.

MODERATOR: So more of a personal choice, okay.

EQUALIZERS2: Just being lazy. Like I tell myself I'm gonna go run in like twenty minutes and then I sit in front of the TV for like another hour and I'm like okay well now it's time to eat something. And I keep putting it off, and I'm just like well now it's ten [o'clock], I guess I won't go running anymore, like [I'll] go do something else.

Later in the focus group, Equalizer1 returns to the feeling of being bored and eating because of that feeling. She also eats when she is stressed and feeling pressured. This group felt a lot of pressure (see chapter 1).

From the Romantics, we find a similar response from one of the participants who said, "The things that keep me from eating right are the sweets that taste so good. And exercising, it feels better just to lie on the couch and watch TV. Especially when I am bored." The Distrusters echo these same feelings:

MODERATOR: Would you describe yourself as being healthy?
[long pause] Anybody?

DISTRUSTERS2: In between.

MODERATOR: In between? So, what do you mean by in between?

DISTRUSTERS2: Sometimes I don't exercise all the time. I just like to eat. I just stay in the house and watch TV and talk to my friends. So, I would be in the middle.

MODERATOR: In the middle, okay.

DISTRUSTERS1: I'd be in the middle too. I eat things, you know, healthy foods. That's about it.

DISTRUSTERS3: I'm sort of [healthy]. I exercise though. I don't eat junk food all the time.

Other groups also used the term "in the middle" and "in between" to describe their relationships to food and exercise as wavering between healthy and not healthy. This sense of being in the middle is an important frame for this group at this stage in their lives. They have a sense of what to do but find it difficult to follow through. They see themselves as teetering between twin challenges including food and exercise. They are bored and watching television or hanging out on the Internet. Like many adolescent girls, they have a slightly adversarial relationship with food. Overall, they do not see themselves as healthy.

One way we can think about these responses is to imagine that they might hold an internal unrealistic picture of health. In other words, to be healthy is imagined as being someone who is always eager to exercise, who is always motivated to eat a certain way, and who never struggles with deciding whether to choose a donut over carrot sticks. We can only speculate here about what is driving those self-perceptions. They may also have developed these ideas through media consumption. And, of course, they view these as personal failures, not as other structural forces at work.

Perceptions of Mothers' Health

Thus far, this chapter has explored what daughters have learned about health practices from their mothers and how that shaped their understanding of health, so we now turn to the ways they perceived their mothers' health. Overwhelmingly the focus groups, except for the Romantics, did not perceive their mothers as healthy, though a few individuals in several groups did. They did see their mothers as resilient, strong, competent, and capable, but not healthy. Perceptions of mothers' health often invoked a discussion of the pressures their mothers faced.

As noted earlier, there were two extremes: the Loners and the Romantics. The Loners were a group that didn't think much about their health, unanimously did not define themselves as healthy, nor defined their mothers as healthy. In contrast, the Romantics, who defined themselves as healthy, were the only group where the majority of individuals unanimously defined their mothers as healthy. For them health was intertwined with being a powerful person in the world and their mother taking care of them. When describing their mothers as healthy, they usually pointed to the fact that she worked out or "ate right," "ate salad," and "she don't eat a lot of junk food."

Other groups were split about perceiving their mothers as healthy, including Equalizers and Distrusters. The Moderates stressed outward appearance as evidence of their mothers' being healthy:

MODERATES3: And, she makes sure that she tells you what to do.

MODERATES2: She makes sure that she takes care of stuff. She makes sure to set the example to always like smell good and always look good no matter where you go.

MODERATOR: Anything else?

MODERATES1: Um, my mom gets her nails done, her hair done all the time. And she dresses nice, like she won't leave the house looking busted or whatever. [Everyone laughs]

MODERATES2: She tries to eat healthy as well and she's outspoken and if she doesn't think that something's right she's gonna politely say what we should do.

There were very few responses from individuals that enthusiastically defined their mothers as healthy. When groups described their mothers as unhealthy, they often pointed to lack of sleep, taking care of others so much that it puts themselves at risk, lack of exercise or inconsistent exercise, and struggles with food (e.g., eating junk food, eating irregularly, skipping meals, or not eating anything). This also mirrors how mothers describe their challenges with health. Food and weight, as I have demonstrated, show up again and again.

The Equalizers' answers to the question about their mothers' health, a chorus of no's and a few yes's, ring out.

EQUALIZERS2: Because she goes to work out, at least once a week. She's a doctor so she generally eats right, isn't sick.

MODERATOR: [Addressing another respondent] And then you said yes as well, is there a reason why?

EQUALIZERS3: Like she said [Equalizers2], my mom does eat right and my mom exercises, she walks every morning and she keeps me and my dad on track.

MODERATOR: Okay, and then you also said no. I heard some no's in the room. Why would you say no?

EQUALIZERS1: My mom doesn't get enough sleep sometimes and, she does eat right, but sometimes she doesn't eat at all.

Tensions occasionally arose about how mothers and daughters were communicating when discussing their perceptions of their mothers' health. One of the more vocal young women in the Equalizers stressed that her mother's attitude was not healthy: "Oh, OK. The attitude. Yes, Check the attitude. Check." She elaborated:

> OK. You know how I was talking about earlier about, like, your demeanor and how you carry yourself? Well, sometimes parents forget that they're setting an example for their children. So, they kind of tend to—how can I say this without being disrespectful? They tend to get—say stuff that they wouldn't want us to say. Yeah. And then once we say it, they get mad at us and they forget that they're supposed to be the ones setting an example. And I kind of feel like that's unhealthy; not just for the parents but the child also. And sometimes they eat bad or they might drink stuff. So, this is just with any family. And then once they find their kids are doing that, "Oh. You can't do that." But you're supposed to set the example.

The moderator noted that there were a lot of "mmm-hmms" and asked people to elaborate. No one else did except the speaker above, who reiterated her points. A similar sentiment was expressed by a participant in the Distrusters.

Many of the girls discussed their frustrations with their mothers' uneven approach to health as related to food. They spoke of their moms' diets and the frustration of not knowing when that would change or when they could and could not eat certain foods. One of the daughters in the Distrusters recounted a trip to McDonald's. She was standing in line with her friend and her mom. Earlier she said that her mother had just begun a campaign of "being healthy":

> So, we just started—normally my mom would have gotten the fries herself probably, so we in the line, we been in the line for a minute . . . She like, "Get out the line." She just started talking about fries ain't healthy, and all that stuff in the middle of the line. She eats fries and stuff all the time. She used to eat them all the time.

This mirrors the mothers' contradictions and challenges. In the previous chapter, I raised the degree to which mothers struggled with a sense of staying on track given demands of work and home life. It is definitely reflected in these narratives by the daughters.

Girls identified positive patterns of health their mother engaged in that could be described as emotional and mental health wellness, or "taking care of herself first, then everybody else." Going out to exercise or to a concert, signaling when things are too hectic at home or at work, and changing one's situation stood out for the girls as examples of this emotional wellness. They used words like "deciding" and "what she wants to do" when talking about the ways they saw their mothers as healthy. Two Romantics shared what made their mother and grandmother healthy.

ROMANTICS1: My grandmother, well, I'll start with my mom. My mother, she's always there for friends and family and if they need help finding a job, she'll go out and get applications for jobs and stuff. Or, like, I had a friend who had a baby when she was real young. And so she helped her to take care of the baby 'cause the mother didn't want to do it and stuff like that. My grandmother, she acts like she's 28! [laughter] And she—I'm serious. I'm dead serious. And she's involved with family and stuff. My aunt was trying to move to New Jersey to do [celebrities'] hair but she has a son. So, my grandmother kept my little cousin, for like two months while his mother moved in up north. And right now she's got some of my cousins are living with her. So, she just—if you need something, we just ask her and she'll try her best to do it. But if she can't, she'll say she's sorry.

ROMANTICS3: My mother works for an organization. And they help people, like, senior citizens. If there's something wrong, they can call up her job and they'll help them. If there's something wrong with their house, they'll get them help. And my grandma, wherever she goes she'll help somebody. She sees somebody in need, she'll help them. All my family members live together in the same area. And my grandmother lives down the street, directly down the street from my cousins. And my cousin just got a new job. So, she has two young kids and my grandma watches them usually for her so she can go to work 'cause she can't find a day care because it costs too much right now. So, my grandmother will help anyone who needs it.

There are some implications from this section that are important to note. Despite the fact that the groups of Experts and Revealers were composed of more health-care practitioners compared with other groups, this did not translate for the daughters into perceiving themselves or their mothers as healthy. This also did not translate to better quality or frequency of conversations or demonstrations of health between mothers and daughters. Yet, given the overall negative evaluation of their mothers' health, I argue that this evaluation constitutes an external and invisible barrier for the girls.

Trust and Daughters' Health

It is important to discover to whom daughters turn to for health advice, where they gather health information, and how they understand the health-care process. Their mothers actively gathered information from the Internet, medical websites, and through other experts. The daughters similarly relied on health information from a wide variety of sources. They talked about searching the Internet but also cited television shows and specific networks, including the Discovery Channel. Even music was cited, as some participants felt that it provided guidelines for how to act in the world, especially related to sexual experience. Media allowed them to double-check what others, both peers and adults, told them.

For health advice and information, they talked to friends and consulted other family members besides their mothers. Teachers and counselors were also identified as people who could give them health information. One participant from the Equalizers explains why she identified her teachers as an important source of knowledge:

EQUALIZERS4: Yeah, this year, now that I have a health and PE course, I've learned more than what I knew before. Now that I'm in middle school, they'll break it down for you, so it's kind of like easier for you to understand what they're actually talking about.

Mothers were not often mentioned as daughters' first choices of consultants for health information and advice. More commonly, sisters, aunts, fathers, and grandmothers edge out mothers' influence. In three groups, grandmothers were mentioned as health sources either because their age made them appear wise to the daughters, or because they saw them as healthy, sometimes as healthier than their mothers.

Trust is a theme that emerges around gathering health information and, more important, seeking health advice. The daughters across groups discuss how they make decisions about whom to trust depending on what the decision was and when it was to be made. The Loners and the Distrusters are two groups that help define the challenges many daughters have around trust and communication. These two groups experienced strained relationships around communication with their mothers. The most striking example were the Loners, who stated that they did not go to anyone for health advice. They did not seem to understand why they might need to. The Loners, as noted before, unanimously did not think of themselves as healthy and were split on defining their mothers as healthy. They were not able to identify people in their life to go to for health advice. They also unanimously did not rely on their mothers' advice when contemplating important decisions except for health-related ones. Instead, they relied on cousins, friends, and themselves. This is also a group that has a high distrust of doctors, as we will see in the next section.

MODERATOR: Who do you rely on for advice about your health?
LONERS1: I don't ask for advice from anybody.
LONERS2: Me either.
MODERATOR: You don't ask for advice?
 Other participants agree and say no in unison.
MODERATOR: We have all participants saying they don't ask for advice.
 [Note taker confirms. "That's right."]

In contrast, the other groups were all able to identify people that they would and did ask for advice about health. What is interesting is the place where mothers figure into this picture. For most groups, again they were not central to the discussion:

MODERATES2: I trust my mother too, sometimes. [All the girls laugh]
MODERATOR: OK, but so why do you go to your sister specifically to ask advice about health?
MODERATES2: Because she'd been through stuff during her age so she know stuff that I'm going through.
MODERATES5: Some things that a mother won't know.
MODERATES6: Sometimes it's easier to ask a sister because they're closer to your age.
MODERATES5: Yeah, or somebody who's been through it before.
MODERATOR: Okay, and you said you like to ask sometimes your aunt, sometimes your mother. So why?
MODERATES6: Sometimes I don't ask my mother, so I go to my aunt, she's like twenty-something, so I ask her.
MODERATOR: So your aunt's kind of closer to you in age, too.
MODERATES1: I don't have any brothers or sisters, so I go to my friends, they're like my brothers and sisters . . . and they're closer to my age. Like sometime like your mother like she tells you stuff that she wants you to do, but like your friends they'll tell you like regardless, like 'cause mom she's like well you need to do this because that's what she wants you to do, but your friends will tell you like the truth. So that's why I go to my friends, 'cause I don't have any brothers or sisters.

The perception that mothers provide information, but often at a cost that is about a specific agenda, and that friends and others will be more open and honest, is shared across the groups. Sometimes girls made decisions about who to trust because of age. For example, the girls cited having similarly aged friends or a younger aunt who was helpful, or a grandmother who they viewed as wise and responsible:

MODERATES4: Most of the stuff that my mom tells me she got it from my grandma, so I would know. 'Cause like I heard my grandma say some things so many times, so it's kind of like alright, I'll pay attention.

Here the Romantics discuss who they go to, and we see a similar pattern emerge despite the fact that they have the strongest sense of their health and were more likely to view their mothers as healthy compared to the other groups.

ROMANTICS1: It really just depends on the question. Some questions I rely on my mother [for advice] and also some questions, my dad. Sometimes I call a friend.
MODERATOR: So you talk to either one of your parents?
ROMANTICS1: Yes. About certain things. [Says with emphasis]
MODERATOR: Certain things. [Laughter in the group] OK.
ROMANTICS2: I kind of talk to my older cousin about most and all things 'cause I look up to her a lot.
MODERATOR: How old is she?
ROMANTICS2: She's 15. I can't go to my friends 'cause they talk too much so I go—or if it's a tiny thing, I might go to my mother.
ROMANTICS3: Me? My mother or my God-mother.
ROMANTICS4: Well, first I will go to my aunt because we're like sisters. So, since my mom had me at a young age, she always was there for me and stuff like that. So, I can ask her anything. She's 25. And then after that, I'll talk to my God-mom, her mom or my other God-mom. And then I'll talk to her [points at girl across the circle] and then my God-sister and then . . . And then I'll talk to [points to another girl] and then I'll go to my mother way after that.

The other two groups, Distrusters and Equalizers, exhibited similar patterns where mothers were consulted but were not always high on the list. This was true even for questions about general advice.

We might have expected to learn that mothers play a more influential role. One reason to explain why this finding was the opposite might be that developmentally, girls are in a transition period from child to young adult. Many of the girls in the study were ages 12 to 14. They are shifting from relying on adult figures as authorities to their peer groups. This is especially true when we look at sexual discussions in chapter 5. Perhaps because the daughters do not view their mothers as healthy, they are less likely to approach them for information and advice. But there is also another reason.

Trust was an important factor in many of the daughters' decision-making processes. Many of them expressed that sharing the most important things with someone can come at a cost. In some instances, the daughter's trust has been violated previously, often by her mother. Other girls did not prioritize their mothers in the decision-making process because when they had come to them with health questions, it had sometimes turned into unwanted conversations about pregnancy and sex. Now, some of this might be explained by developmental factors, as I alluded to. The consequence, however, is the same in that if some girls are less willing to go to their mothers for specific kinds of advice, this creates less motivation to seek help navigating relationship and intimacy choices.

What is striking and important is that the person(s) the girls view as trustworthy for providing health advice will also be the person(s) that they transition to for advice about sexuality. This is what we will learn in chapter 5. Daughters' decisions in one area of life in seeking help tend to have a cascading effect in other areas. And, we will explore the contrast between daughters' perceptions about how skillfully their mothers communicate about sexuality with how mothers view themselves.

Health Providers and the Medical Encounter

There has been little attention given to African American girls' experiences with health-care providers and face-to-face experiences.[2] Young people are observant, sensitive, and may pick up cues in a medical encounter that are overlooked or downplayed by adults. What are their perceptions of health providers? How do these girls experience their health providers, and what do they think of them? What is the culture of health that is being understood by these girls? We asked girls about their experience of health care, what they liked and did not like, as well as how often they saw someone.

The daughters were raised with some form of access to doctors and medical care and saw general practitioners, dentists, and podiatrists on a regular basis. Some girls who have chronic health conditions have seen specialists. Some did have uniformly negative experiences with providers, most notably the Loners and Distrusters. The Moderates were concerned with the possibility of the threat of inappropriate touching and said that they felt disrespected by doctors. On a few occasions, girls describe positive experiences with providers. Most other encounters were neutral to good.

We begin with the Loners. One of the Loners says flat out that she does not like the doctors that she visits. The moderator probes:

MODERATOR: You don't like them?
LONERS1: I have no feelings for them. [she pauses]
MODERATOR: Go ahead. [encouragingly]
LONERS1: I don't like them at all because I feel like they're not there really to help you. They're doing a job . . . because, first of all, I really need to go into detail—my grandfather was in the hospital for a whole year and the nurses did not take care of him like they should have. And I lost my respect for nurses because they slack off on their jobs just so they can get paid well. They don't really talk—well, that's not all nurses. But for the most part, I have to get to see their character, you know, know them for myself. But I feel like they're not there for you. You know how people always say stuff is confidential? [Others nod] The nurses would tell you whatever you tell them was confidential. They would go in that little work room, workshop, whatever you call it and talk about you just like a teacher, just like a teacher would. Yep. That's why I feel like that.

Loners1 added that they typically do not "go to the doctor" and that when they do go, they try to "get in and get out." At the end of the exchange above they added, "I'm just being honest. I do not like it. Do not like it."

Here it is possible that because the daughter perceived a negative situation with her grandfather's care, she has formed an overall negative evaluation of nurses. It is also important to note that due to this experience and possibly others, her desire to see a doctor is low.

Two others in the group felt that their treatment by doctors was "good." And then another girl said:

I agree with that. It's OK, but I don't really go into the doctor's office to make friends I guess. [Laughter] I might need to get a prescription or something.

The Distrusters had an equally engaged discussion about health providers. One of the participants felt strongly that in one instance, a physician's assistant did not listen to one of her concerns about her son bumping his head and the resulting injury that it might have caused.

DISTRUSTERS1: And, they won't write it down. And they're supposed to. So I just tell the doctor and I guess they'll talk to that person. But I don't know. Sometimes I just tell them. I keep on telling them 'cause they never find the right answer. [agitated]

MODERATOR: So, how do you feel about that?

DISTRUSTERS1: It's disrespecting me. I'm telling you about a problem before it's too late and you're not doing anything about it.

After expressing more displeasure with her son's doctor, this participant was asked about her experiences beyond her doctor and the medical system as a whole:

> It's OK. It could be better . . . The first thing . . . [when a patient arrives] make sure that they feel like you're—that they should listen, that you're not just oh, off in another world and never hear them.

Another person chimed in and said she did not like being asked "crazy questions" and perceived it as "for you to know all my business." The moderator said, "So when you say, 'crazy questions,' like what? What's a crazy question?" Distrusters2 answered quickly: "Like they ask you, 'When's the last time you had sex?' Your period and stuff like that." Another person quickly responded, "Like they your mother."

Agreement converged in the group. There was discussion from the first person (Distrusters3) about being asked questions that should be in the chart and others in the group. Distrusters3 added, "And, it's like they pressure you to tell them. But if you don't, they'll try to guess it and figure it out. Like, if you don't need to know, don't try to figure it out 'cause you're not going to get it."

There was some discussion as the moderator tried to determine the demarcating line for the participants between health-care providers getting essential information and then crossing the line of being disrespectful or even "nosy," as one of the girls labeled it. They did differentiate and noted that sometimes it is important for the doctor and nurses to ask specific questions, especially if sexual assault was involved. They also said it was fine if doctors asked questions if you tell them a certain body part is hurting (e.g., breast tenderness). But, the majority of the group affirmed that doctors and nurses asked them questions that seemed "nosy" or out of place.

In the Moderates, the topic of not being treated well was raised in response to the question, "How do you feel about how doctors or nurses treat you?"

MODERATES4: Well from watching TV, like this is my opinion from watching TV and hearing like what the doctors do in the clinic and so many crazy things goin' on in the doctor's office. And when it comes to the time when I do go to the doctor's office, I make sure my mom does not leave the room just in case, because you don't know if you can trust that person or not, and for me growin' up to be my age now, like I'm more mature to know what's wrong, what's right, what people would do to me, and like to know that if they put they hands on me then I would know what to do in that kind of situation, that's why I don't trust people that I don't know.

[The conversation continued as people agreed with this speaker.]

MODERATES5: I agree with her. As long as my doctor continues to treat me in a professional manner than we're okay, but as soon as the line's crossed then—

MODERATES1: —I know, that's right!

MODERATES5: —Then I'm not going to go to your office anymore and I might have to file a complaint if it's that serious.

MODERATOR: Have you had experiences where doctors cross the line and don't treat you professionally like they should?

MODERATES: [All] No.

MODERATES4: But I've had some teachers do that to me, but it was like when I was younger and I didn't know much, but now when I think about it it's like you know that's really messed up, that's wrong.

MODERATOR: So give me an example of what would be professional or what wouldn't be professional.

The person could not follow up with a specific example, but instead talked in generalities. And then Moderates4 gave the example of "groping and touching." She goes on to say:

MODERATES4: When I watch TV you hear about the doctors that do things to women that take away their identity and self-confidence, when I think about it . . . you went to school to go be a professional and this is what you do?

Moderates1 responded to this comment by talking about being aware of one's surroundings when in a doctor's office. She also noted that one of her family's personal friends is a doctor and she feels comfortable talking with her informally. Finally, she added that she feels more comfortable with a female doctor and her mother always stays in the room with her. As the conversation progresses, they talk more intensely about gynecologists, male versus female. They almost all agree that they prefer and trust female doctors over male doctors. Moderates3 stated that when her mother goes to see a physician, if she is assigned a male doctor, she always requests a female provider to be in the room. One person notes that women can be unethical as well. Moderates4 agreed and offered insight into what her mother had shared:

My mom got a checkup a couple of weeks ago and she said that she would rather have a male doctor than a female because when it comes to the point where that doctor crosses the line, she said she wouldn't want it to be a female 'cause that's like weird. She said it's most common for a male to do something like that, but [with] a female it's not like that, it's not the same thing.

What can we make of these different instances in which several girls have impressions of doctors being disrespectful, not interested in them, or too interested in them? The Loners and Distrusters, as has been established, are groups that express a low sense of health and well-being; they typically do not view themselves or their mothers as healthy. The Distrusters' mothers are the Transitioners who were actively managing their health. The Distrusters tended toward a more skeptical worldview and also had other negative experiences of health. The Loners' mothers are the Revealers, who also had a high level of dissatisfaction with health-care providers. One of the Distrusters is a mother and has not had positive experiences working with her doctors. We can only speculate whether her experience with providers results from the intersection of her racial background, her status as a young mother, and her socioeconomic status. Given what we know about the prevalence of racial and gender bias for African American patients, we should not necessarily be surprised that some daughters' experiences were negative.

We might want to say that their experiences can be explained by age and the emotional development of the girls, that doctors and nurses have to ask probing questions in order to receive useful information, and that girls may feel that they have little control in that exchange. That is possible. But for daughters, this theme of respect and even trust echoes back from earlier sections that extends to other relationships. The feeling of not being listened to by health providers was also mentioned in chapter 2, by mothers.

For the Moderates, in keeping with their overall worldview and orientation, several people had formed impressions from TV and media. It was interesting that their opinion and concern about inappropriate touching was formed from TV and not in actual experience—this speaks to the power of media. They made the connection to other people with authority and power over them, for example, teachers. It is unclear if Moderates4 was also talking about or making a reference to inappropriate touching by a teacher. This issue did not reemerge later in the conversation, so there is no way to know for sure.

The fact that some girls across groups anticipated being disrespected when accessing health care is troubling. We tend to minimize young people's experiences with providers. This encourages more work on how Black girls interface with the medical system. What is striking in the overall pattern is the finding that few girls had positive comments or stories to share about their providers. This should lead us to pause and rethink ideas about how Black girls experience health care. One possible outcome of these daughters' experiences may be a reluctance to seek medical care when they are adults.

Conclusion

These narratives reflect contemporary challenges for young people in the twenty-first century, including a lack of consistent physical activity and excessive access to junk food. Health was an emerging and somewhat precarious concept for many of the girls. The focus groups converged on thinking about health as broad and malleable. The idea of health was also linked to mindset, which included faith and spirituality.

Health for many daughters was understood as being physically and morally clean. There was a strong emphasis on being clean and having a robust hygienic regimen that, for many girls as they are approaching menses, receive strong and consistent messages about the upkeep of their bodies from intimate others. There is little specific intersectional work on girls of color and menstrual experiences. One study found Black girls were underprepared for their menstrual cycles in comparison to white girls (Scott et al. 1989). However, the daughters here did not seem to be underprepared or harbor negative feelings about their bodies; "being clean" was naturalized (of course, it would be this way) regarding menstruation. Might this hyperfocus on being clean influence how the girls view their maturing bodies? Could a hyperfocus on cleanliness alienate them from their bodies? Could these messages about cleanliness be a component of how some Black girls experience young girlhood?

Several girls linked confidence to health and healthy practices, which suggests that there is an emphasis on being able to stand out, express oneself, and take care of one's "business." Health was also connected to other responsibilities that were gendered, including "taking care of a family."

Only the Romantics uniformly thought of themselves as healthy, with the majority also describing their mothers as healthy. Health was something that many daughters believed was within their control, but they were often unable to make their individual efforts related to diet and exercise stick. Like their mothers, they face internal and external barriers to maintaining their health. In discussing barriers to health, they have often internalized the more acceptable and popular notions of restraint and self-control. The challenges around food and exercise mirror their mothers' health challenges. Taking a broader lens, the other factors that may be at play are less easy to see and include structural challenges like mothers working two jobs and the perceptions of their mothers' health as negative. The girls have access to health information and often turn to people close to them, but have strong feelings involving who they will trust with their most important decisions. Their challenges provide a mirror to the mothers' health challenges. If they do not view their mothers as healthy, they are less likely to go to them. Who you trust determines who you get advice from, and given that many daughters are wary of their mothers because of an erosion of trust, this may have a cascading effect as they mature. This is especially salient given that health and sexuality are intertwined in the minds of many of the daughters.

4

"I Want That First Kiss to Be Perfect"

Mothers on Intimacy, Pleasure, and Sexuality

In this chapter, the primary focus is African American mothers' reflections on their communicative strategies with their daughters about sexuality. What is important to mothers to communicate? What is difficult? How do they navigate daughters' resistance to their communication? Participants wrestled with their daughters' transition, moving from the protected space of girlhood to young womanhood, when they will be interested in dating, relationships, and sexual experiences. In listening to how they narrate their experiences, we are able to witness and understand the challenges they perceive. The themes in this chapter reveal the threats they viewed to their daughters' transition into young womanhood. These include combating negative peer influences, male attention, and popular culture influences.

I took up questions of intimacy to understand how mothers thought about their daughters' future choices, but also to veer from a traditional focus on sex, which has often meant surveillance for African American girls. There are few spaces for African American women to discuss intimacy. This aspect of the conversation offered the mothers a unique opportunity to discuss with other African American women the nuances and complexities of raising a daughter.

Mothers' communication strategies with daughters as they relate to intimacy revealed just as much about their own complex relationship histories. This thread of the conversation catapulted them into memories and emotion. A thread of deep regret, grief, and even cases of acknowledged trauma were expressed throughout the groups. These emotions were most often expressed by women who were parented by a young mother (sometimes a single mother), who themselves began parenting at a young age, or who are single parents. Several women have overlapping membership in these groups. In many of the focus groups, especially the Strategists, members shared their distresses and at times comforted and counseled each other.

Pregnancy was also an important and charged conversational gateway. Many of the most intensive moments in the focus groups about their communication with their daughters was talking about pregnancy. This encompassed both fear of their daughters becoming pregnant and challenges with their own pregnancies. Pregnancy was viewed as a derailer. The mothers articulated that an unplanned pregnancy for their daughters conflicted with the future aspirations (especially educational) they held for them.

We turn now to explore the concept of legacies in mother and daughter communication and how mothers either borrow, incorporate, or reject communicative styles and patterns from their mothers.

Legacies

"I'm Not Like My Mother, I Talk about Sex"

Mothers often wanted to distance themselves from their mothers and/or grandmothers who they characterized overall as having a lack of knowledge about health and sex and an unwillingness to disclose what they did know about sex. This was a salient theme throughout all of the focus groups. Mothers had a tendency to characterize themselves in opposition to their mothers and grandmothers regarding health-care access, sexual knowledge, and openness of communication. The terms they most often used to describe their mothers were prudish, unhelpful, and hostile. They said that their mothers often talked in euphemisms when it came to sex (e.g., "don't let boys go under your coattails"). Many mothers discussed at length that their mothers and grandmothers were ignorant of or extremely conservative about sexual information.

For the few women who were able to have some communication about sexuality with their mothers, many said that it quickly turned to concerns about pregnancy. The Revealers demonstrate this pattern:

REVEALERS3: As soon as your period started, it was not about hygiene. It was about you could become pregnant now. Hello? My period, I had my period five minutes ago and we're talking about getting pregnant and having babies. That's my only conversation I had. Something about [keeping] the corners of the knees [together], whatever the heck that is. People would put coins—[laughter] [Cross-talk about keeping one's legs closed like holding a coin]

REVEALERS1: So, it was not discussed.

REVEALERS2: [Agreeing] Not at all.

REVEALERS3: But I was always such an open person about sex and my body that, you know, if I had something down there I was like, "Ma, what is this? Here's a flashlight—look." She told me about my period. That's about it. But when it started, I took my underwear, "what is this?" [Laughter] You know, and she was like if you don't get your drawers out of my face.

REVEALERS1: Yeah!

Revealers3 repeats that she was always an open person.

REVEALERS2: It was taboo.

REVEALERS3: But I'm always open. And then when I decided to have sex for the first time, which was very traumatic, I thought I was never going to have sex again. I went to my mom before, with my little pill pack in my hand and said, "Mom, I'm ready to have sex. I got my pills." You know, she was, I'm sure she was screaming on the inside. But I was mature enough to go to the doctor, get my pills and then I went to her. And, you know, she never mentioned it again; never asked how I was or anything. But I've always been so open with my body and sexual functions that—but my mama didn't tell me squat. So, I don't know where I got it from [her openness in talking about sexuality]. I have no clue how.

This was a common experience across all the groups. Lack of sexual knowledge and discussion of sexuality among some African American mothers and daughters is not uncommon. Alexis Dennis and Julia Wood interviewed 20 African American college-aged women and asked them to discuss remembered conversations about sexual communication with their mothers.[1] They found that the majority of daughters could not recall a lengthy or sustained conversation about sexuality with their mothers. Mothers, in the focus groups, also recounted negative messages and feelings of discomfort when talking about sex with their mothers. They considered their mothers as important role models and expressed a desire to have gained more knowledge about sexuality and relationships from their mothers. Other research also supports a historical pattern of incomplete and insufficient communication between African American mothers and daughters.[2]

The women attributed their experiences to the fact that African American women three to four decades ago experienced great financial distress and challenging social conditions. Their mothers had to cope with the effects of de facto segregation and the Jim Crow era, and they had to deal with other stressors related to racial oppression and sexism. The majority of the mothers stated that without proper information about their bodies, they were often disadvantaged when negotiating heterosexual relationships. They expressed regret, anger, and grief about the lack of conversation around sexuality and sexual health. This was common across all focus groups but was particularly true for mothers who became pregnant at an early age. These mothers in the Experts provide a good example:

EXPERTS1: I told my older sister, when I first had my first period. I had it at school and I was scared because I didn't know what it was. So nine years old and I'm

going eh! So I go home, I'm going Ma! Ma! And she's going "Yeah, I gotta cook and I gotta do this" and I'm like no, we gotta talk. We go in the bathroom and I go what's this and she goes oh. She grabs a tampon and she says here, use those and now don't let little boys under your coattail, and out the door she went.[3] And I was like, coattail? I was grown before I ever knew what a coattail was and I think my husband had to tell me because I didn't understand. I said, well my child's not going through that, that's scary not to know and your mother just goes mm, mmm, yeah, it's alright. I had a child at 17 and that's because my mother never talked to me . . . she just assumed I knew it, go ahead, maybe you'll be alright later. And it doesn't get alright later. Now I'm happy, but I'm free when my daughter comes to me and she's like, I want to ask you something, but I'm scared and I'm like, "get over here and talk to me!" And she's like ah! It's OK, come to me, talk to me, talk to me, I want that relationship with you because my mother (and I) did not have that. Oh my goodness, it [sex] was a bad word you just never spoke it, body parts were just mm-hmm. "Just get it together," and that's the most she'd say and I'm like (makes sound), that's not gonna work for me. Now I've got two girls, so I gotta talk about something! You know I can't just sit, I've got an 18- year-old son and two girls, I gotta teach them better than what I was taught. Because I didn't get anything. Now my sister, I'm very envious of her because she got it [some conversation about sex], but there's nine years' difference for us, so by then my mama had time to mellow out and say, well this is what's going on and dadahdahdah, and my sister goes, "Well, we had a wonderful conversation!"
[All delivered emphatically]

This comment is reflective of similar discussions across focus groups. Notice the pace and intensity of language of this respondent's narrative. The mother positioned herself as a proactive communicator with her daughters and son because of her negative experience with her mother. The following is an example from the Strategists:

STRATEGISTS2: I told her, I want you to wait [to have sex] until you're in a relationship, married, you in love and all that stuff. And I said if it's something that you feel that you just have to do, I can't stress enough, please come to me to make sure that you have the tools you need to do this. I mean, and I say it, if you can't come to me you better go to your aunt, you better go to somebody. Because in this day and time, you can prevent a lot of things, so you just have the knowledge not to just, of course I don't want to hear it, I don't ever want to hear her say, "Mom, I did it! But . . . I know I'm sorry."

STRATEGISTS6: My daughter, she told me everything, the things that she was telling me there's no way I could have told my mama, none of the stuff she was telling me.

STRATEGISTS2: Well, that's good because I couldn't tell my mama some of that stuff, the conversations that me and my daughter have. I went to my mama and asked, "Mama, do you think I could get? [birth control]—No! You get birth control you gonna be having sex." But I wasn't! I was not, but I knew I was gonna be leaving home and I knew I should be prepared. And she was like no, and I could have gone behind her back and done it. And I said no, she said not to do it. Well, I took him home, I didn't set out to do it, but it was too late! . . .

When I finally went [to the doctor] it was, they gave me some pills. And I never took a pill because I was [already] pregnant. [Everyone laughs]

STRATEGISTS6: I never talked to my mother about birth control. Never. I ain't never talked [about sex] to anyone other than to my sister.

Interesting to note that Strategists6 echoed the comments of other mothers—they talked to female siblings about sexuality because they could not talk to their mothers. This was not an uncommon disclosure among the mothers. The extended conversation below between mothers in the Nostalgics group highlights how they talked about intimacy. The mother said she found some notes written by her daughter that seemed to indicate her daughter's friends were feeling some pressure to have sex. Her daughter and her daughter's friends are 13 years old:

But, OK, this is a conversation her girlfriends are having. Some boys pressuring one of the girls and, you know, there's this dialogue going on. And I can't act like I know. But when I think of intimacy, I guess I do think of sex. And even though, you know, my mother never had conversations with me [agreement by other women], I mean never. It was never, there was no dialogue. There was only, once I started menstruating, "OK, now, you can get pregnant and you better not get pregnant or I'll kick you out." And I understood that very clearly. And so part of my dialogue, talk with my daughter, unfortunately or fortunately, is no babies. I'm not raising [her] to have any more babies. I've got two, got the two. I'm done. No baby is coming. And I verbalize that. "There's no babies." "Oh, mom, that's not even"— you know, she's in total denial. But, I know that's part of it, that there are conversations about sexuality going on with her peers. And I would love to say that our relationship is such that we've had real frank dialogues about what you do and how to protect yourself and all that. But it's not there. Every time I approach the subject, she goes into denial.

Or, like "I don't want to talk about that. I'm not"—but my whole thing is you're going to keep hearing from me. No, unprotected sex. I'm also saying to her, I don't want you to have babies, but I'm not in total denial about the fact that her hormones are raging and, at some point, she is going to have sex. And so I'm just like, OK, you've got to protect yourself, you've got to be aware. You've got to take control. So, when I think of intimacy, I think I really want my daughter to control her interactions and not make the mistakes that I did, or just giving in to peer pressure, you know.

Their mothers are invoked in these narratives as prudish, difficult to speak with, and unable to provide the kind of support that the mothers needed as adolescents. Because of the desire to distance themselves from earlier mothering practices, the mothers in the focus groups also tended to portray themselves both as "health- and sex ed-savvy." This meant that many mothers indicated the myriad ways that they distinguished themselves from their mothers in that they actively discussed sex, "watched Lifetime and music videos" [with their daughters], and "got on the Internet to educate themselves" about sexual issues.

Talking about Intimacy

When designing questions about how mothers perceived their daughters' sexual development and communication around that phenomenon, I and the research team were intentional with use of the term *intimacy*. We felt that it was important not to hyperfocus on sexual practices as that was already well-presented in the health literature. By using the term intimacy, we were aiming to learn how they thought about potential relationships for their daughters and the representation of relationships in popular culture. Questions about intimacy were used intentionally to create space for mothers to speak to both the mundane and aspirational ideas they have for their daughters, to ruminate on best- and worst-case scenarios. The groups varied greatly in how they approached and thought about intimacy. Creating intimacy for the mothers meant acknowledging their own and their mothers' limitations. They talked about strengthening that bond between them and their daughters to prepare them for what is ahead in their development. Sometimes the conversation shifted quickly from intimacy to sex even when the moderator used the word intimacy. That might have been because it was easier for some participants to discuss their concrete concerns regarding sexuality versus more abstract ideas about intimacy.

Questions of intimacy are the trigger for a mother's disclosure about being born to a young mother or being a young mother and/or single parent herself. The discussions about intimacy raised tensions among mothers and sometimes created distress in the group, which was evident from the body language and decibel levels of the participants' voices. In this section we pay attention to the Strategists and the Experts. They tended to be at the opposite end of the spectrum in how comfortable they were in discussing intimacy with their daughters.

The Experts had the fewest challenges and greatest ease in talking with their daughters about intimacy. They did not express the same fears as many of the other groups. They also expressed the fewest regrets sharing their own experience and stressed disclosing information about their relationship choices to their daughters. Conversely, the Strategists exhibited high levels of distress in talking about intimacy.

EXPERTS3: As far as being with . . . guys? Or just? [sighs, others laugh nervously] well we talk all the time, because I'm a single parent also. I mean we sit down at the table so I know everything that's going on. [With] some things she might be, "You might get mad about this," and she'll say it anyway, both of them, even my 9-year-old. And that means a lot to me because I really didn't get to do that with my mom and like what these ladies are saying about doing things with them to make them feel special, that's something I'm big on because I didn't do anything with my mom and I think that is an issue for me today. Not having that bond. I feel like it's so important to have that bond, that mother-daughter, my mom and I don't have it. I think she's trying to get it now because I've moved away.

Experts3 then talked about moving away from the area where her mom lives and answering people's questions about how could she have moved away from her. People often asked her why she does not live closer to her mother, especially as a single parent:

It was very easy [to move away] when you don't have that closeness and I think it's because she had me so young. At 15, she was still a child, um, and everybody around her helped some. She was my mom, but you had this person here doing this, this person here doing that, so she had responsibility but she didn't [have it], like I have. I had my daughter at 18 and I just feel as far as me knowing who she is, regardless of what she may go out there and do, she knows what I tell her and the experiences that I had, because I really don't hold anything back, um, neither does their father. We're just really open with them.

This speaker went on to state that the bond between mother and daughter is important. She referenced her previous comments about how her bond with her daughter helps her talk about health issues; she believed in the power of listening to her daughter, a seemingly simple act that for her yielded positive results. She did not have an open line of communication with her mother, nor did she feel as if she was listened to. She contrasted this approach by stating that her mother would have "knocked me out" for the kinds of questions her daughter feels comfortable asking. She reflected that her mother did not have the time for honest and open communication and is now trying to make up for it "a little too late." She acknowledged that her mother having her at a young age, along with excessive work demands, were factors that interfered in her mother's ability to be there for her. For this mother, establishing a close bond was also the key for talking to her daughter about everything, including health.

Later in the group discussion, another mother commented on what she has shared with her daughter about intimacy:

EXPERTS2: I think I'm probably too comfortable, I think for her comfort. But for me, I always tell her this is not my job to make her happy or make her comfortable, my job is to make her a good adult. And part of that is, I had her very young, I was a freshman in high school when I had her, her father is four or five years older than I am. And I said you know I believed everything he told me and that's one of the things I try to stress with her, in a relationship, not one person should be in control of anything. And like that's one of the things that I think intimacy-wise is still something I try to stress with her, because if a young boy wants to be intimate with you, you shouldn't be intimate with him because you're afraid that he might not like you.

This mother elaborated and said she also was not ready to be a young mom, but she adapted and "rolled with the punches" and the life situations that she found herself in. She was a young mother and did not have all of the facts she needed. She stressed that this life experience is what motivated her to speak with her daughter early on about sexuality. She felt that doing so was of the utmost importance:

So you know it's sort of one of those things, when I talk about intimacy with her it's much more in a sort of power [and] control issue and her being in charge of making that decision, like that's something that you want to do and if it's something that you want to do, like my mother, my mother's whole birds and the bees talk was "it hurts, don't do it." I mean like, that was it from beginning to end—it hurts, don't do it. And so I've tried to sort of say, you know Bridget, it

[sex] doesn't hurt, it feels good, and it should feel good and it should be healthy, but it should be something that you do with all the knowledge and in the right circumstances and in the right places and with the right person, and right is your decision, I'm not going to make that decision for you. But, think about it, don't do it because, oh my friends are doing it or I saw it on MTV. I mean there's a lot of stuff that they kind of just get in and for me it's trying to tell her that it's so important who you're with and who you give your body to.

Experts2 refers to her expertise as a health educator and explains what she envisioned for her daughter:

Because I'm a health educator I've tried to give her the facts, like use a condom, I don't care what he says. I was a teenage mother and people I guess saw me as a success, I was able to finish high school and finish college and now work on a graduate degree, people are like oh you were successful, so I feel successful, so I've had a chance to talk to other teenage girls who, they always laugh at me because I always tell them the same thing, you tell a boy that the only way he's gonna have sex with you is with a condom. He's always gonna choose with a condom. You do that with any boy and tell him the only way he can have sex with you is with a condom, he will always pick the condom! Rather than not have sex, trust me, I know, I've tried it! I've run my own little experiment here! And people always laugh at me because it is really that simple, you have to take control of it. So, I sort of preach to her the same thing, I tell other teenage mothers that I talk to, that it really is about choice and power. And you should enjoy it (I'm not approving it), but it should always be because you want to and not because somebody else says you should.

This mother brings up issues of power, control and also, importantly, pleasure. The concept of pleasure was absent from the majority of other mothers' discussions of intimacy. Only one other mother across the groups discussed pleasure and not feeling guilty for sexual desires, and she was in the Revealers:

But I really want to be able to talk with her about what love really is in relation to having sex and be able to have it make sense to her so when she does fall in love, she won't feel guilty. It all comes from something in church that you're made to feel guilty. And I'm like, "I don't want you to see sex as something nasty. It can be something beautiful." I wish I knew how to communicate that.

Experts felt very confident sharing their insights with daughters and tried to provide good role models of loving relationships. Experts1 noted that she has a very loving relationship with her husband, which presents an important model relationship for her daughter to see, one that is not abusive or a "hollering and screaming match." She also discussed some of the challenges of making the decision to have a child at an early age, but this decision is not laden with any regret. She stressed that it was important "to never lie" to her daughter "about anything." She leaned forward while speaking and spoke quickly, as if entranced. She shifted from speaking to the group to addressing her daughter. In the excerpt below, she recounted her life decisions as if recounting a story, one directed at her daughter:

> I had your brother when I was 18 years old. It wasn't the smartest decision, it wasn't the dumbest decision. I just had him and if I would have known things that I know now I would have done some things differently, but I didn't do that. I got caught up thinking, hey he loves me, whatever, you know. What he's going to tell you today is not going to be the same thing he's going to tell you tomorrow when all is said and done. With wisdom and age, I was able to distinguish crazy talk from real talk. You not getting that right now, he's going to say anything in this world, yes you are built like an hourglass, he's ready, he's going to follow you, ooh aren't you pretty, ooh can I get, ooh my goodness, and he's going fill your head and it's going to balloon like this [spreads hands apart].
> [Delivered with intensity]
> But, I credit myself with helping to bring that balloon back down because I tell you the same things. You are pretty, you are a sweet girl, you are an individual who desires, who wants things, who needs things, and you can get all that stuff and it doesn't have to come with the price of you laying on your back to get it. And you didn't ever see me laying on my back, you don't see men running in and out the door all hours of the night, you didn't see things like that and that's what I expect from you. . . . I expect more from you. . . .

The speaker went on to say that her daughter hates to talk to her about sex (maybe because she's embarrassed), but then goes on to state that she and her daughter do talk about sex:

> I want to keep that line open so if you got a question like that, you feel comfortable enough saying it in front of me, you might regret it because oh Lord we're about to talk about sex . . . And we talk about things. I talk to her friends about as much as I talk to her, you know because I didn't get that and I wanted to be the total opposite of my mother, I want my house to be welcoming (to her and her daughter's friends), I want you to feel like you can talk about any of that.

And if it's sex we gotta talk about, then sex it is! I don't care where we are, we'll talk about it because I'm excited you came to me and asked, you know because you could've gone the other way and decided not to. That's how I feel about that.

The Strategists show a similar pattern of discussion and revelation during conversations about intimacy. Notice here, too, how the single-mother status is raised:

STRATEGISTS6: I just talk to 'em like . . . try to make her get an understanding, talk to me like you talk to your friends.
STRATEGISTS5: Try to get her to open up.
STRATEGISTS6: Yeah, open up, don't be afraid not to talk to me about anything 'cause when something goes wrong you gone come to me anyway, I gotta take you to the doctor right, so you better tell me what's going on now! [Everyone laughs]
STRATEGISTS4: What I've found, say, with the friends things, they talk more openly if their friends are around. So sometimes if her friends, they're over, I just kind of pop in the room . . . they'll tell me things and I'll tell them do this and this, and I think it's good. I guess they feel more pressure when it's just one on one, you know. Feel like they been put on the hot seat.
STRATEGIST2: Yeah, I tell my daughter all the time, you know I love you and I would not have done it any different, but I don't want you to have to struggle like I did to raise you by myself, that's not fun. I don't regret it, through the grace of God and my family, my daughter has not had to want anything but, I just think how, would her life be different if her father was around. We just had a discussion the other day: Well, do you regret that your father's not here? And she said, "Well, of course I think about him." But she made me feel good because she also said, "Mama, you're doing a great job." And I just got all teary! [Everyone laughs, someone says, don't cry!] I'm just worrying, you know. So we talk about these things always. I mean she's almost grown, I say thank God, but then I worry all over again, oh she's gonna be out there in the world, she ain't gonna have me to go to. [Everyone laughs and nods sympathetically]

Talking about intimacy often led to a discussion of their fears and what I call "derailers" for their daughters. This theme is discussed in-depth later in the chapter. Their focus is on pregnancy, but also in many instances it's on sex before marriage. In conceptualizing how to discuss intimacy with their daughters, the Revealers make a point that is echoed in other groups—that having their daughters discuss romantic relationships (with them or others) is OK, having romantic feelings is OK, but they do not want their daughters to get caught up in the "fantasy of sex." They perceived that the fantasy of sex is represented as engaging in premarital sex without the potential consequences of contracting an STD or becoming pregnant and is driven by popular culture:

REVEALERS1: You know, I said to my daughter, "just wait till you get married. Just wait till you get married." Now, she was watching this movie called *Love and Basketball*. I don't know if you've seen it [group reacts, some agreeing]. [Cross-talk] She was literally watching that movie a hundred times. She says to me she needs something to make her go to sleep at night. She watches that *Love and Basketball* over and over and over and over again. But I stress to her, I said "[to my daughter], they still are having sex before marriage."

And I said, "You don't want to go away to college and come back with a baby. You know, they didn't [in *Love and Basketball*], but it could happen." And so those are my two concerns; the sexual abuse and sex before marriage. I just don't want those two things to happen to her.

The above Revealer mentioned sexual abuse as a concern. This was a concern among some mothers, but not discussed in-depth in comparison to their other concerns.

During the discussion of intimacy, there is recognition and agreement among mothers across groups that their daughters are in the middle of a major transition, navigating new emotional territories:

STRATEGISTS2: My thing is it's hard for me to accept and realize that she's not a baby anymore. When she was 14, I was still trying to hold her hand when we were walking. I always made her walk on this side of the street so the car would hit me and not hit her. . . . it's just a mother thing, baby girl. She says, "But I'm not a baby."

[Someone asks: How old is your girl?]

STRAGETISTS2: She's 16.

STRATEGISTS6: Two more years and technically she'll be a woman.

STRATEGISTS2: Oh yeah, she's graduating next year!

STRATEGISTS6: Alright!

They worried about how their daughters will manage their first serious relationship, particularly a romantic relationship that may become a sexual one. They wondered what would happen to their daughters if that kind of relationship goes badly. This rumination triggered their memories about early relationships. An example from the Revealers is illustrative:

REVEALERS5: Another thing that I worry about with my daughter too because she's so sensitive is, you know, that guy who's telling you well, I love you, I love you. Let's have sex. And then that day he doesn't call and he's not interested in her anymore. You know, just kind of keeping her from having that broken heart.

REVEALERS2: But you can't protect her from that. [Agreement and cross-talk]

REVEALERS5: I realize that. After I broke up with someone I loved, I stayed home from school for two days and I stayed in that bed. And I remember how I felt. And I do not—and that's what we all try to do, prevent from going, from hurt—to take that pain away from them.

REVEALERS3: That's really scary to me.

Discussions of intimacy reveal how mothers grapple with their excitement about their daughters' entrance into a new life phase, but also how it can remind them about their own romantic pains, rejections, and disappointments. These memories haunt the primary narrative that revolves around their daughters. Almost all of the mothers had spoken with their daughters about some form of relationships and intimacy. Although the term intimacy itself was elusive, the broader idea of sexuality, sexual contact, and relationships was salient. While in Strategists and Experts, reflections about their own experiences tended to dominate and overshadow the discussion of their daughters' issues, other groups were mixed. One could argue that when the focus groups were conducted there were different stakes involved for the groups. The Experts' daughters were younger than other groups, daughters were just approaching or not yet in puberty, so it may have been easier for the Experts to project aspirational futures for their daughters. However, overall, as a group they were more comfortable talking about sexuality.

The Strategists responded differently. They had many more fears about what might come up for their daughters. Some Strategists pushed themselves to talk with their daughters. When asked, "What does it feel like to share with your child some of the more difficult or even traumatic things about one's own sexual experiences," Strategists6 responded that it allows her daughter to learn and be open to new things. She also repeated in her narrative, "What I went through, I hope she doesn't go through."

Being a young mother, feeling as if they could not talk to their mothers about their sexual experiences, being a single parent, and/or being born to a young mother were the most important markers of identity for the mothers participating in this conversation and were launching pads for disclosure of their own experiences as young women. These experiences drive and shape the prism through which they see their daughters and what they will share with them. Overall, these patterns tended to push mothers in the direction of frank and open communication with their daughters. As we shall see in the next section, these mothers also paradoxically seemed to use the most intensive strategies communicating with their daughters.

Communicative Strategies

I Put the Fear of God in Them

Mothers employed several communicative strategies in discussing intimacy with their daughters. Much of the communication mothers reported with their daughters around intimacy and sexuality was related to virginity and what not to do. The mothers' exclusive emphasis on intercourse and virginity as the defining markers of sex, sexuality, and sexual interest was a primary focus. In many of their discussions, mothers focused on wanting to prevent their daughters from having sex, which was overwhelmingly defined as genital heterosexual intercourse.

Despite their desire to represent themselves as being more open than their mothers and trying to establish communication about relationships and intimacy with their daughters, many of the mothers admitted to searching their daughters' bedrooms for evidence of sexual activity. This is a representative statement made both by mothers who had their children at an early age and who were currently single parents. This mother in the Transitioners group just finished telling the group that she had recently searched the room of her 17-year-old daughter, and some of the other women reacted with surprise:

TRANSITIONERS1: You know why I do it? Excuse me (to another focus group member), I'm going to tell you why I do it and tell you why I'm actually like I am . . . because when I was coming up, a lot of other things I do now with my child my mama didn't do with me. Because if I really had that mother . . . My mama was just the opposite.
[Cross-talk]
TRANSITIONERS1: If I really had that mother and daughter talk and stuff like we really should have had, maybe I wouldn't have had a baby.

The Strategists also spent some time elaborating on their fears about their daughters' potential sexual activity:

STRATEGISTS6: I was letting her know, just because you might not get AIDS, but they got herpes out there. She was like—what is that? So I say you better get

into these books girl, you better start reading. I'm telling you about a lot of different things that you probably don't even know about. So you better think two
or three times before you think about just laying down with a boy, don't look at
it like just because he got a Trojan on you're going to be okay. 'Cause that don't
work no more. And she talking about, "for real?" For real! I got her scared!

STRATEGIST3: Well my daughter, with my daughter I just throw the fear of God
in her. I have her babysit her brothers . . . her brother's 13, he has ADHD, and I
have a 7-year- old, now both of them running and playing and actin' crazy!—

STRATEGISTS6: She's like uh-uh!

MODERATOR: How old is she?

STRATEGISTS3: She's 15. And she's just like mom, no, and then she babysits on the
side also. She's like "kids are throwing things," and she's like oh my god! And
then she's the choir director of the kids' choir at church, she's like "Oh my goodness." She said, "This is it, right?" [Meaning this is how kids act] She's just scared
now. I mean, I didn't try to per se scare her, but it's just like she's involved with
a lot of stuff with kids, like younger kids, and she's getting a feel for it, she's like
uh-uh, no. She likes looking at other people's babies, she can handle that. But
she's like, "Mom, right now I'm not ready for any of that right now."

MODERATOR: Okay, so we're talking about like making sure that they know what
the consequences are for engaging in sex too young. Has anyone had the opportunity to ask your daughter?

STRATEGISTS5: If they're a virgin or not?

MODERATOR: Right, or about that specific conversation?

STRATEGISTS6: Yeah, I did it.

STRATEGISTS2: Are you sexually active? No? Are you kissing? [Others laugh]

STRATEGISTS6: Yeah, because you know kissing leads to other things.

STRATEGISTS2: I told her, you know, boys is something that I want you to wait
and not do until you're in a relationship, married, you in love and all that stuff.
And I said if it's something that you feel that you just have to do, I can't stress
enough, please come to me to make sure that you have the tools you need to
do this. I mean, and I say it, if you can't come to me you better go to your aunt,
you better go to somebody. Because in this day and time, you can prevent a lot
of things, so you just need the knowledge. Of course, I don't want to hear it, I
don't ever want to hear her say, "Mom, I did it!"

[Cross-talk]

As noted in chapter 2, HIV/AIDS is not a strong focus for the mothers.
HIV/AIDS makes an appearance in these discussions, as do other STDs including syphilis and herpes, but they are just noted and not fully explored;
the recurring narrative thread is pregnancy and virginity. In many of the

exchanges, mothers often reinforced each other's comments about the importance of virginity (often in the context of marriage), by leaning in, lots of nodding, verbal cues of "that's right," and laughter, which in this case was interpreted as both familiarity and agreement. From mothers' narratives in the focus groups, they primarily engaged in scenarios with their daughters about what not to do. They also provided strong narrative indicators that there were "good girls" and "bad girls" (clothing was mentioned extensively as markers of behavior), and that they wanted their daughter in the first category.

My Daughter's Listening (to Me), But Is She Really Hearing Me?

The participants stressed that in contrast to their own mothers, they talk to their daughters significantly more than their mothers did with them about sexuality and relationships, and they use more direct strategies. Some strategies involved passive listening, being around when their daughters' friends were over, and acting like a fly on the wall. They also tried to answer their daughters' questions when asked. More common strategies were for mother to initiate discussions with their daughters and seemingly force discussions. They often took the approach, "I'm going to make you discuss these issues." Their daughters, to their recollection, often resisted these conversations, but that was not always viewed as a problem. They talked about forcing them to have the conversation or talking at them. The mothers said that daughters often employed avoidance strategies with their mothers, saying, "Not now, mom," or "I don't really want to know." In recounting these situations, mothers offered that they did not let their daughters' resistance stop them.

Several mothers across the groups talked about the tangible benefits of discussing ideas openly with their daughters. They were laying the groundwork for thoughtful discussions later. They often came back to the stark realities of not being able to have engaging and informative conversations with their mothers about these topics. The Experts, as in other areas, approached their discussions with their daughters in pretty optimistic ways.

EXPERTS1: Now I don't think she's reserved in coming to me, I think her sense is if I ask mom, she's going to get real excited, because she's got a whole lot of knowledge and really wants to give it to me and I really just may not be ready for it [speaking of her daughter]. You know because I may overstep, she may just say, "What is herpes?" and I'll explain and then I'll add something about syphilis, and she says, no mom, "I just said herpes I didn't say nothing else." [I'll say] Be quiet, I just want you to know everything. And she'll just walk away, but

I don't think it's because we don't have a good rapport, or that she's fearful of coming to me, I think it's that . . . she's just not feeling hungry for a whole lot of conversation right now.

EXPERTS3: Don't want to be lectured right now.

EXPERTS1: Yeah, mom's going to get the slide show out and the books [all laugh]. So no, I think, personally I think she's a little, this is my personal opinion, I think she's happier that I'm that way as opposed to not being, because it's like, when she started her period I prepped her for a year, this is what's going to happen, this is what your body's going through, you know this is what you have to do, this is how you have to wash. . . .

Experts1 goes on to ironically express how surprised she was at how nonchalantly her daughter behaved when she got her period. She had been preparing her since she was nine, so she realized that much of what she said was sinking in because at 14, her daughter was asking good questions and was not shocked. She talked about the importance of getting her daughter ready:

I want to prepare her early. I don't want her to be caught out there and have to try to figure things out on her own. She needs to understand about breasts coming, she needs to understand her hips widening, she needs to understand pubic hair and underarm hair, and smells and all this stuff. She's got to understand that and who better to teach her, but me? I didn't have any of that stuff, so I'm telling her and yeah, at nine, it may have been a lot, but now it's kinda like . . . she does her own thing, she's aware of things and she keeps herself the way I told her, and I'm very proud of that.

Toward the end of this thread of the conversation, Experts1 stressed her belief that her daughter will feel more confident around both boys and girls because of the knowledge she has been given about her body.

For some mothers, this way of directly engaging their daughters helped them lay a good foundation for what they wanted their daughters to know and encouraged them to come back and ask questions. They saw their daughters' reluctance as natural. They also felt some urgency to be aggressive in their approach as they knew their daughters were part of larger community conversations about sex and relationships. As one person in the Experts noted, she knew her daughter was "listening to everybody's problems [of a sexual variety] in the neighborhood." One Strategist said she does not sugarcoat anything, whether her daughter likes it or not. She said that her daughter's friends also come to her for advice about relationships: "They still keep coming back over and over, so I think I'm doing something good."

A Transitioner mother discussed the importance of talking to daughters about peer pressure. And, some of the impetus for communication, reiterated here, is if they don't speak with their daughters, the daughters will find information out from other kids. Mothers expressed concern that another child will be "more advanced [sexually] than your child." How to handle information that their children get from peers and school frequently came up in discussions. This mother from Nostalgics described what she hopes goes through her daughter's mind when her daughter is thinking about being sexually active:

> And I know you're going to think you love or trust him. It won't be the first and it most definitely won't be the last. You will have many loves over your lifetime. Trust me, you will. This is not the end all, be all, do all. So, don't put everything into one situation. You just have to be careful and you have to know. And then of course in this day and age you could die from one night of SEX [Inaudible]. So, you have to look at all of that and you have to really look at the person and how they're treating you, how they feel about you, what kind of relationship you have together outside of laying down . . . I hope my voice is there when she comes to make that decision. [and I want her to think] Maybe I should wait. It's scary.

Nostalgics1 echoed a similar sentiment:

> It's something that you have to be prepared for. And it's more than just your body. You have to be prepared in your mind. You have the rest of your life to do that [have sex]. So, let's take this thing in steps and let's focus on what you need to concentrate on first. I'm always saying, you have the rest of your life to hang out with girls. You have the rest of your life to play and blah, blah, blah. Do what you're supposed to be doing now and take steps because, again, I'm not trying to be raising no children unless they're my grandchildren; and ideally, the same way as my mother used to always tell me, "Well, yeah, I want to be a grandma but I want the son-in-law first," and blah, blah, blah.

There was a sense among some mothers that because they employed many of these strategies of communication, they were well informed about their daughters' experiences and preferences. The conversation in the Transitioners group highlights a common pattern of mothers' understanding of their communication with their daughters. One mother said, "I talk to her about everything, so I already know." Another mother agreed with this statement. In the Strategists, an interesting moment emerged in their discussion about listening and how to tell whether their daughters are truly hearing them and absorbing the messages the mothers are sharing. This is also from the group that searched their daughters' rooms:

STRATEGISTS2: She wants me to be quiet [joking about this comment]. She says, not again please! Especially not about the little boys. Nothing! Do we have to have that talk again? Please!

This respondent later commented about watching her daughter interact with her friends and believed that her daughter was "being a leader and not a follower." Peer pressure, she said, was also a motivating factor:

STRATEGISTS2: Peer pressure. So that's what you really gotta talk to 'em about, don't let no one tell you to do nothing that you don't want to do, don't let no one try to make you do something that you don't want to do. I don't care who they is.
STRATEGISTS5: 'Cause most of their friends will be more advanced than your child.
MODERATOR: Most of their friends are farther . . . ?
STRATEGISTS5: Sexually active.
STRATEGISTS4: But you know what I've found too is that you can be naïve and think that our child doesn't know or is not . . . they talk about it at school, they know more about it than we do.
[Other women are vocalizing their agreement with "um-hums."]
MODERATOR: So what is that like, when you want to talk to them and you have so much to give or to have this discussion and their attitude is "again"?
STRATEGISTS6: Mine don't tell me that, they know not to tell me again, they are going to sit there and listen. I don't care how many times I tell you we need to talk, she listen.
MODERATOR: Do you feel like they're listening?
STRATEGISTS6: I know the difference when she is listening and when she isn't.

The mothers mostly believed that what they were saying was well-received by their daughters. They reinforced each other's ideas. In several of the groups, however, the mothers also wrestled with what was the right amount of communication. They struggled with the questions: How much is too much? And, when is it enough? They asked each other these questions and counseled each other. Some mothers recognized that although they were actively communicating and doing so in more diverse ways (through popular culture, one on one discussions, etc.) than their mothers, they were not always sure what the right amount was. After the moderator raised the question about their daughters listening, the Strategists delved into the topic further:

STRAETGISTS5: If they listen a lot, if they really, you know, are they telling you what you want to hear. You really can't tell, I mean you really can't tell.

STRATEGISTS2: Yeah, if you look in their eyes when you ask them things.

STRATEGISTS6: But I feel, to a certain extent, by me talkin' to her, in a way I know if she is telling me a lie and if she is telling me the truth because the way, it depends on how close you is with your daughter, and how you talk to her and the same, the way that she do it, the way that she say it. And then when you say things to her about certain things . . .

STRATEGISTS6: The expression she get, is she gonna cry or say, mommy I'm telling you the truth, I wouldn't lie to you. You will know if she is just brushing you off. I let her know, I was a child just like you was so you can't get nothing past me . . .

MODERATOR: Are you ever concerned that you are either, um, giving too much information or not enough information? That you're unsure of what the balance is? In communicating with your daughter about certain things?

STRATEGISTS6: I don't feel that way.

The mothers talked about finding a balance. Some did not express concern about finding a balance, but others did:

STRATEGIST2: I do sometimes because, I don't want overkill, but then I don't want to just sit back . . . if I feel like I gotta say it whether she thinks it's overkill or not. But sometimes I don't want her to just tune me out because it's like [her daughter is thinking] she's still talkin', still talkin', we already had this conversation ten times. I mean, my thing is I'd rather say too much than not enough. So I guess if I'm not balanced, I'm giving too much information. But I think about it.

STRATEGISTS4: I think our role as parents is to inform and I think sometimes we think they don't need it when they really do, because sometimes the kids at school will tell them what they know when sometimes they don't know and they give wrong information. So I encourage my daughter, okay, so if it is something you need to know, you need to come to me. Please.

A little later, Strategist5 sharpened her comment to what was her main concern.

STRATEGISTS5: Is she really listening? Is she thinking, oh mom, "she's always talking." [Delivered emphatically]

STRATEGISTS6: That's why, even if they won't talk, that's why you show her different things so she can see—

STRATEGISTS5: I mean, she could be listening but then what they do out in the world is totally different.

STRATEGISTS6: That's why you got to get her to see things.

[Talking over each other]

STRATEGISTS5: That's just a way of life for them, you know? You know, that's what everybody's doin', I ain't gonna be left out. Everybody's picking on me because I ain't doin' it and blah blah blah. Boys pick on you, girls pick on you.

STRATEGISTS6: 'Cause they like to be accepted.

[Agreement by others]

MODERATOR: Is there anything that you can think of that might ensure that they're listening, that you would do or that some, some practice that you think might work better than others, like a video?

[SOMEONE SPEAKS]: Lock her up in the room with a doctor.

[SOMEONE ELSE SPEAKS]: Right, give her a multiple-choice test.

STRATEGIST5: Yeah, just write down some questions and then she gotta pick whatever four answers. Hand the test back to me and then say all this is wrong, look at this! And tell her.

STRATEGIST4: I actually took mine to the OB-GYN and I didn't go into the office with her. I let her go with the doctor. She was an African American doctor and they specialize in informing teens and she went back and gave her some information. The doctor came back out and talked to me and said, I'm gonna give her this, this, and this, is that okay? And I said, "Tell her whatever you want to tell her, I want her to be informed, I want her to know everything. I think I told her everything, but I don't know everything. Tell her everything, everything you know, tell her!" And she took that time and my daughter really liked her. And, you know what she said? "I learned some things." And, I said, "That's what I wanted."

This mother involves another authority, a doctor, to support her communicative strategy. The Transitioners also employed this strategy. Transitioners2 was one of the two mothers that commented at length:

Not yet because, you know, I even, believe it or not, you might think I'm crazy. But I asked her, "Have you started having sex?" She said "Mama, no!" You know, the reason why I do this is because I want to know. So, a lot of times if I feel that she really ain't open with me about certain things, I'm gonna tell you what I will do. I make a doctor's appointment and I allow them to tell if she's still a virgin. Because he deals with kids.

From these communication strategies, we can observe the following methods and concerns mothers expressed: (1) Mothers tend to feel empowered with their choices and in helping their daughters deal with the pressures they faced from popular culture and peer groups; (2) From their own experiences, they have seen what happens when there is little to no communication; (3) They use a variety of strategies of talking about issues related to intimacy; (4) Most often their daughters do not choose the timing of their mothers' discussions about sexuality and are required to listen; (5) Often their primary concern is to prevent pregnancy and to keep their daughters as virgins for as long possible.

Virginity was highly valued among the mothers. In analyzing these patterns of communication, one sees that there is little opportunity for daughters to choose the timing of discussions, and that much of the communication is often adult to child. Daughters must listen and many mothers believe that they already have significant insight into their daughters' questions and how to navigate young womanhood. Again, we have seen that this is more pronounced with single moms and working parents. Additionally, despite the confidence that some mothers portray about their repertoire of communicative strategies, they also used outside authorities to confirm their daughters' virginal status and, as demonstrated with the Strategists, they wrestled with their choices. For mothers who began parenting at a young age or who were also single parents, discussions about intimacy triggered a discussion of regret in recounting their own sexual histories.

Daughters' Derailers: Pregnancy, Gendered Peer Pressure, and STDs

Mothers described the kinds of situations and people that they considered to be harmful and to potentially derail their daughters from a healthy lifestyle, educational achievement, and economic advancement. Their three main fears for their daughters that could derail her are pregnancy, contracting STDs, and what I identify as "gendered peer pressure." As stated earlier in the chapter, an unplanned pregnancy for their daughters was a primary concern for the mothers. One of their central goals of communication with their daughters was to stress the importance of delaying sexual contact for as long as possible. Pregnancy was considered a derailer that diverted time and energy resources away from finishing high school, attending college, and pursuing future aspirations that they held for their daughters. They were generally disturbed by and felt strongly about the wide-ranging cultural acceptance of teenage pregnancy and the educational accommodations made for it. They also expressed skepticism about abstinence policies and how these policies ultimately placed more responsibility on them in the home.

Late into the conversation, the Strategists discussed what kinds of situations might cause their daughters to ignore them and their advice. As the topic emerges in other focus groups, the mothers likewise express concern over peer pressure and how that leads to poor decision making and can lead to pregnancy as well as other challenges. This participant states the opinion that kids want to "be grown" and will follow other people's lead, no matter what you tell them:

> Girls want experience. They want to go through it and when they get to that point, even though that's your only child you hate for them to go through it, but when they get hot headed and they don't want to listen, sometimes they just gotta go through it.

Right before this reflection, another mother discussed how kids are susceptible to peer pressure and they sometimes don't want to listen to common sense. The moderator asked this mother if it is her perception that kids are just stubborn. The participant replied it's about being "hard-headed." Then another mother interrupted, one who had not spoken for many minutes:

STRATEGISTS4: I think this whole generation's different. Because now when young girls get pregnant or whatever, they're proud! I mean they just strut around like it's nothing to it. [several others agree] When it happened in my day you were ashamed, you didn't want nobody to know! I mean you can go to schools and see the young girls walking through, they don't have a problem with it—
[Delivered emphatically]

The conversation moves quickly and all the mothers get involved.

STRATEGISTS6: —It depends on the person—
STRATEGISTS3: —It depends on the school too. A young lady got pregnant over at Viewpoint, which is a new high school and is predominantly white and they have a few Blacks or whatever. She got pregnant, they sent her over to the old high school in the area—Sunrise High [predominately Black]! Because they don't want that interfering in class, they don't want it to seem like they're promoting getting pregnant, so they sent her over to the other school. And at Sunrise they have a day care over there for the kids. So they do it like that.

As the discussion progressed, Strategists4 raised the dilemma of informing other mothers about what their kids are doing according to her daughter's information. They also agreed that if you break your daughter's trust, it is difficult to get it back. As Strategists3 said, "I mean once you're in there, you're in, you're in good." [The mothers agree, everyone starts talking, joking about leaving the other mom an anonymous note.]

The woman who started the thread of girls being "hard-headed" dissented, and at this point said that most girls are not trying to get pregnant and that often girls see the limitations of being a young mother. Strategists2 says some girls are not intentionally trying to get pregnant, it just happens. Strategists6 interjected and made a distinction about what some of the kids are paying attention to:

STRATEGISTS6: But we're not talkin' about the kids that are already into sex, we talkin' about kids that are not even into sex at all who are lookin' at the other kids and the girls who are pregnant, they don't want to be bothered, they aren't even with them. I sit talkin' with my daughter and stuff and listen to the things she says, "Mommy, that girl who's pregnant, we don't talk to her, it's like *a disease.*" [Emphasis added]

STRATEGISTS5: But I think times have changed, just like you said, it's very different.

STRATEGISTS2: And some people might think, well yeah those things are out there but it really ain't gonna happen to me so I can just do it this one time.

Strategists6 agreed with this comment and went on to say that she believes times have changed, parenting styles have changed, and it depends on child-rearing practices. Another mother mentioned that many parents are "working double shift jobs." There is some disagreement in the group about how much attention people generally give to their children. There is some discussion about the challenges of (some of the mothers) working two jobs as well as paying attention to their kids' extracurricular activity. Another mother acknowledged that it is really hard to keep track of all that their kids are doing: "Even when you work a normal job and she's in church!" Strategists3, who had been quiet previously, joined in the discussion and commented on the material conditions that affect her parenting:

But, I'm saying sometimes we get sidetracked! I stay in a neighborhood that's kind of bad and I look at it like this—my daughter and my son's in the house, end of discussion. I close the door, you know what I'm sayin'? That's how I relate to things like that because the neighborhood we in, I'm gonna close my door and I'm through with it. Because long as I know my kids are in the house, they are in the bed or just in the house and I can keep an eye on them and that's it, sometimes we get sidetracked [from the basics], you know.

This comment animated discussion and others directly responded to Strategists6:

STRATEGISTS5: [Turns to Strategists6] I understand, but when you can't keep an eye on them and they're with their friends, that's where the problem is.
STRATEGISTS2: You right, you right.

Strategists6 defends herself and stresses how important it is to know the kids that are spending time with your kids. She also stressed talking to and visiting the parents of your child's friends. The group seemed to minimize Strategists6's comment about how important safety was for her family.

A sense of being overwhelmed emerged as the mothers expressed their lack of control of their children's influences and also the potential undermining of their values while their daughters are at school. To them, all of these things can lead to pregnancy. Strategists6 expressed adamantly that kids can act differently across multiple environments. In the Revealers the conversation has a similar narrative flow to the Strategists about teen pregnancy:

REVEALERS2: The church that I go to, there are so many young, unwed mothers. It's like, it just—
RVEALERS5: There's no shock to it anymore. [Agreement from others] It used to be when we were high school, they were women—
REVEALERS4: They [pregnant young girls] went to a separate school. You know, like, disappeared.
REVEALERS5: Yeah, you know, they didn't come to school anymore. But now at my daughter's school, there's just like [so many of them] [cross-talk]—wow.
REVEALERS1: Every other week.
Yeah [agreement from all].
REVEALERS2: So, I think about last summer—every time I turned around my daughter was like "Yeah, such and such is having baby shower. Such and such is having a baby shower." But after she went to one or two and I thought about it and I said, "Hold up. We need to talk. You aren't going to any more baby showers." She was like, "Why?" She was kind of offended. And I said, "Sweetheart, it's not normal." [Agreement from other mothers] "If you're going to baby showers, you need to be going to baby showers when you're like my age. You know, you shouldn't be going to baby showers when you're like 14."
REVEALERS1: She shouldn't know anybody [in that situation]. [With emphasis]
REVEALERS2: Yeah! So, I was like, "You can't do that because I don't want you to get used to something like that." So she goes, "Mom, you're being judgmental." No, this is just my rule. You don't need to be going to too many baby showers

of somebody's 15- or 16-year-old child." Like you said [points to another participant], it's not the shock of the peer group. [Cross-talk]. Good grief, yeah.

REVEALERS3: But then they make it easy because they can get day care in school and they can get services for free [agreement]. I think it makes some of them just want to do it again. It's so easy.

The group debated about the perceived current ease of accessing services when you are a young mother. Unlike in the first group, however, where the conversation evolved into the different ways that daughters acted in public and private, this discussion was interrupted from that trajectory by one of the participants, who challenged that providing services to young mothers was a bad thing:

REVEALERS5: Well, yeah, and I'm gonna be the devil's advocate on both ends. It's good that they provide that stuff [agreement from some] so that the mother will stay in school.
[Unidentified speaker] Right. That's true.

The participants discuss this issue and there is some general agreement that providing support services to young mothers is a good thing, however, it quickly shifts back to what they see as popular acceptance of teen pregnancy:

REVEALERS5: Yeah, I know. But, I know what you're saying, too, 'cause sometimes the other pregnant girls just make it so appealing.
[Agreement]

Revealers1 continued with renewed intensity:

To them, you know, their life doesn't stop. They come back to school. Their child is in day care. They carry on the same way. They're probably going to do the same thing, they dress the same, you know, they look nice. They look "with it," just like me. And they just have a child at home. And they might even go to the party or to a social . . . So, it's not like it's the end of the world like we used to think [agreement]. Your life stops. You know, whether you're a teenager or no teenager, it's like, you know, they can maintain and they can do just anything that you can do and still have a child. So, it's not like a punishment.

Later in the conversation, this first mother brings up pregnancy again and Revealers3 responds:

And to me it's not good when you go to high school where three-quarters of the girls have babies. I don't think that is good. And it's just like that song that Fantasia sings—"Now it's like a badge of honor to be a baby's mama."—that's what my daughter will say, "Now it's like a badge of honor to be a baby mama." And these kids think that, you know. It is like, "I'm crossing over because I have this baby and I'm young and I'm having this baby." I don't know. I really think these young people need other things on their minds, give them other interests.

At the end of this, the respondent affirmed her desire to communicate with her daughter and talk with her about images she sees in the media. She also disclosed that she had a child out of wedlock and described how difficult that was for her. She says that she shared that with her daughter, asking her to learn from her mistakes in saying, "You don't want to raise a child alone." Even though she was not a young mother, she had raised her children without a partner for some time and she wanted her daughter to understand the nature of intimate decisions.

The Nostalgics echoed the conversation with the Revealers, using strikingly similar examples. One mother discussed being a young mother at age 19 and went on to discuss how tough it was to be a young mother in her community. She mentioned a community of girlfriends who were also pregnant and how her closest girlfriend tried to hide her pregnancy up until the eighth month. She also made a passing reference that there were other girls who were pregnant and had abortions as early as the sixth grade. Others in the group responded to her comment with surprise. There was much cross-talk before it settled down enough so that she could elaborate:

NOSTALGICS2: Yes! Yes. This is why—role play, OK? [reference to an earlier remark about the importance of role playing with her daughter about sexual situations] And so, yeah, so I learned a lot from her and then I was like the third [person to get pregnant] out of that group. And after I got pregnant, they [the adults] started having all these meetings. They was like trying to figure out how they could lock down their kids, you know. It was like a disease! [Laughter] Which was fine for them but it was extremely hurtful for me! It was really hard for me. Like people stopped talking to me.

She explained how the community turned against her and how difficult it was as a young mother to navigate the world without support.

NOSTALGICS3: I find myself sort of debating with my daughter about the fact that it's not OK being a teenager and pregnant. I'm sorry. I don't care what the song is. It's not OK! Because it seems that the pendulum has swung the other way.

NOSTALGICS1: Way the other way—

NOSTALGICS3: When it was so acceptable, you know, to be a young girl and be pregnant, you know. No! In my mind, it's still not OK. And it's not that you're a bad girl.

NOSTALGICS1: Right.

NOSTALGICS3: It's like your life options are just sort of really narrow, you know. So, I think that that's interesting in terms of what's happening in the world of girls. What's normal has definitely changed.

NOSTALGICS1: Yes, because back in our era it was more than the fear of getting pregnant. It was reputation, morals. [Agreement] For me, I was just afraid. Just straight up afraid. That was the farthest thing from my mind at 12 years old. I don't even know if I consciously knew what a penis was at 12 years old, let alone think about trying to have some sex, you know. And then as I got older, I was still scared. Just straight up scared of the act, scared of pregnancy, scared of my mom finding out. There was just no way nobody could talk me into anything. But now, it's a badge of honor. [Agreement by other mothers] It's unheard of to find virgins these days. Now they're starting to talk about it more. "Oh, no. I'm a virgin. I'm gonna remain a virgin." But that's just a slow turnaround because, like you said, it's like—the norm now. [Agreement] [Cross-talk]

We finally return to the Strategists after a discussion of popular culture, and they also reflect a dominant way of discussing pregnancy and parenting:

STRATEGISTS4: Because I'm on a committee, in my county, and we're studying disproportionate minority contact [suspensions in high school]. If you look at the race of students that are suspended, and then drop out of school, it's like almost 80% compared to any other race. Why is that? But a lot of people say that if you look at our race that we have a lot of kids having kids. Like if a 13-year-old-girl had a child, now the child is 13, the mom is 26. So, when the mom comes in to see the teacher, the mom is wearing the skirt up to here and then you wonder why the child is dressing that way. [Others express their agreement] It's because the mom . . . I'm buyin' my child's clothes so she can only wear what I buy. So if you look at it in that way it's almost like, you know it used to be that in church or whatever you would have these old moms who would tell you—you can't wear that! Cover up girl, whatever. And if you look now, we got the grandma out trying to get a man.

STRATEGIST3: Because the grandmothers is young.

STRATEGISTS4: So it's almost like the generations are getting so mixed up that we don't even have the older generation that's supposed to teach the younger, you know how to act and how to respect yourself and if you don't value your body, they're not gonna value it.

Here we have a few points of interest. The mothers, in most cases, perceive the acceptance of teen pregnancy as a break from traditions. They also have mixed feelings about services being provided for teen mothers. Their discussion about pregnancy can be interpreted as a referendum on parenting. They worry about how the influence of peer pressure and popular culture may influence their daughters to become intimate, which can lead to pregnancy. As we shall see later in this chapter, there is a focus in the discussions on their daughters' dress and behavior. The degree to which mothers feel a loss of control is also shaped by the other social and cultural forces of the moment. This can be linked to respectability politics and shifting norms. Respectability politics refers to the ways that societal ideas about appropriate behavior (especially sexuality) and dress for girls and women, across different backgrounds, govern behavior and reactions to them.[4]

Keeping Her Safe: Babies as Deterrents and Brothers as Gatekeepers

As we saw in the previous section, mothers used varied efforts to maintain the virginity of their daughters and also to keep them from becoming pregnant. The mothers employed a wide range of communicative strategies with their daughters. They employed other techniques as well, including searching their daughters' rooms.

One of the other ways they tried to combat threats of pregnancy was having the daughters "exposed" to people with babies or very young children. They also pointed out couples or friends that had a child at an early age and pointed out some of their problems. All of the groups shared a version of making sure their daughters encounter people with babies as a deterrent. Laughter and agreement often accompanied the memory of employing this strategy.

STRATEGISTS2: Then it's just helpful for my children to see the struggles of people with children . . . knowing, okay, this is what happens when you have sex when you ain't ready. It's like, oh, they ain't goin' out all night, they at home with the baby. They can't do anything, they at home with the baby, they can't get any new shoes, they have to buy for the baby! [Others agree]

When this comment arose, another respondent offered a long comment about watching her daughter observe the challenges of child-rearing by watching her uncle:

> She's just like, "Mom, I'm not gonna be like this." I said, "Just pay attention, watch everything they going through. I'm not going to say nothing else, watch them . . . everything . . . the mistakes they're making, things, changes going on, watch them. They are young and not married. So anytime, she could walk away or he could walk away. Just keep looking." We don't do much arguing on that. [Everyone laughs]

The respondent said she reminded her daughter that if she became pregnant, she would not be a constant babysitter. She said she asked her daughter, "What are you going to do when he starts hollering and yelling and you can't shut him up, what are you gonna do?"

Mothers spoke highly of school programs where children were assigned a computerized baby to take care of for a week. They found it to be an effective strategy for reminding their daughters of how difficult child-rearing can be. They often welcomed and encouraged their daughters to participate (if it was voluntary) and cheered them on when it was mandatory for all the children (e.g., in a sex ed class). In three of the five focus groups, women said their daughters had participated in such a program. This Strategist echoed the other mothers:

> Remember they did the dolls in school? I said that's fake, that's false advertisement because in a real day you gotta spend 20, 30 minutes to an hour figuring out what's wrong with that child, you can't put the key in and shut him up. You gotta say, oh I gotta check the Pampers . . . You gotta spend time to figure out what's wrong. I said to my daughter, "So don't ever think you gonna have a baby, put the key in and shut him up. Don't ever think that because it takes more than that, for real!"

Another common technique of deterrence among mothers was showing their daughters babies being delivered. The Strategists talked at length about the ways that they try to expose their daughters to the actual process of childbirth, which sometimes meant watching current popular television shows or encouraging their daughters to be in the delivery room when possible:

STRATEGISTS4: I have an older daughter that's 27, she's married, and she had my grandbaby. So my younger daughter went in the delivery room. And, I told her, "This is what happens when you have sex, plain and simple."

STRATEGISTS2: My daughter has had the chance to see a birth because of the program she's in at school.

[Others jump in talking about watching births.]

STRATEGISTS4: They all need to go!

STRATEGISTS6: Mmm-hmmm. Now I let my daughter watch it on TV, let her see that's what happens when you have sex.

STRATEGISTS2: But, it's nothing like being in the room there.

Strategists6 shares that her daughter has also seen a live birth on TV. She talks about having open lines of communication with her eldest daughter:

"I was just like her best friend," and how that was a successful strategy that she is trying to implement with her youngest daughter: "I try to be open with her and let her know I'm your friend, not just your mother. I ain't going to harm you."

After discussion back and forth she adds:

Then I got a son who's 23, *he stays on her too*, so. [Emphasis added]

Mothers employed other strategies to discourage or prevent their daughters' interest in sex and avoid pregnancy. The last line in the quote above helps lead into the next observation. Brothers and other male figures besides fathers (i.e., uncles) played a key role in how several mothers managed their fears about their daughters' potential pregnancy and how they kept track of their daughters' actions outside the household.

The terms for these men who kept track of their daughters included helpers, surveilers, and enforcers. The phrases "stay on her," "keep track of her," and "keep an eye on her" were common refrains. This meant they encouraged various men in their daughters' lives to be aware of the young men they expressed interest in and to monitor the girls' friendship circles. They also had license to monitor a girl's dress and/or public behavior and sometimes intervene with their daughters.

These male figures were mentioned by daughters in the focus groups without much affection. Indeed, as we will see in the next chapter, the girls were quite resentful of male siblings and others, specifically because of the way that they treated them. The girls often saw this treatment as unwarranted, sexist, and controlling. Only two daughters said that this strategy was effective.

Girls Today: Gendered Peer Pressure

Mothers' fears coalesced around the impact of certain kinds of peer pressure that other girls could exert on their daughters. Other girls' behavior and the potential of that behavior to impact decision making for their daughters was a primary concern. They criticized other girls' dress and behavior as problematic. Some mothers were worried that if their daughters followed the trends of how some of their friends dressed, they could be perceived as older and more mature than they were. One participant said she worried how kids, and in particular how girls, dress: "My little daughter, with [wearing] these tight jeans and the way they can dance and move their bodies. We got to keep up constantly and check on them." Another person in this group affirmed, "That's true. That's true."

They were less worried and animated about the boys in their daughters' lives but were rather more worried about other girls. They seemed resigned about boys' behavior.[5] Boys were described as having a universal and unchanging nature, possessing the same kind of characteristics and aims that defined the boys that mothers knew in their adolescence. They often described boys and young men in animalistic terms.

A grandmother in the Revealers, after identifying that she talked to her granddaughter about sexuality as portrayed in videos and also in song lyrics, went on to explain how she views male behavior. This quote is representative of the sentiment across the groups that boys want "one thing," sex, and "will say and do anything for it." And, boys can be clever and use "sweet talk," and in the end it is never worth damage to one's heart or one's reputation. Girls implicitly carry the responsibility of morality:

> And I said [sex and the way that's portrayed] that's the gut-bucket. That has nothing to do with intimacy. And while we were having this conversation this little dog from the neighborhood started hanging around the house. And she [my granddaughter] wants me to mate the dog with our dog, which I'm not going to do. But she kept talking about him hanging around and started saying he was our dog's "baby's daddy" [laughter]. She went on to say, but "Mom, they'll have such nice puppies. Do you think he would still come around and check on the pup?" It's not like that with dogs! It's, you know, a dog's in heat, he smells, he comes, they mate and that's the end of the ball game. They don't get married or think about goals. [Cross-talk and agreement.] However, with humans you make a conscious decision because you have free will over your mind and your body. And you can make a conscious decision of what to do and what not to do. And I'm talking to her about guys [that] will say and do anything that they have to get you to drop your

drawers. And then after you do, they'll talk about you like a dog. They may still be around for a while. But ultimately you'll be the one that's stuck with the pregnancy for nine months and then I'm stuck helping you to raise that baby, you know. You've got to look at all that. You've got to trust them. You've got to know a person.

But, in many mothers' estimation, girls are a major concern because of how they dress and their influence in popular culture. In mother narratives, "other" young girls are consistently presented as more sophisticated, more assertive, more difficult, and having more advanced sexual knowledge. Across groups, these characteristics were universally discussed. This Nostalgics captures the way most mothers viewed their concern about other girls:

NOSALGICS1: But what scares me is other young girls who are more mature for their age, usually just in body only. But—and I know that my daughter is— well, she's 13 and I don't know what is mature enough for 13. But I don't think she's that mature in my eyes because of her actions and the way she looks at things and the way she talks about stuff. I think she's still a little girl. And these days they just have so much to deal with at such young ages and just the boundary between the 13-year-olds, when you've got a 13-year-old that's looking 10 or acting 11 and then you've got 13's looking 21 and acting 31. And, you know, what scares me is associating with some of those girls and perhaps wanting to be like those other girls, emulate those other girls in spite of what you tell them.

Moving to the Strategists, one of the more talkative participants said that she started a church group and that it has allowed her to be privy to conversations with many young women. She stressed to the other women that "it's different now" for girls and that there are more chances for girls to "get in trouble" and for other girls to influence girls to make bad choices:

I mean it's different. The information is there if they want it on the Internet, with friends in school, on the bus, I mean they're gonna learn so many things that we can't even, I mean they tell you things and it's just like I don't know even what to comment. They even know that's not right to do but everybody else is doing it, and in the end, you know, they're getting along fine, it doesn't seem like anything's happened to them. And I mean, it's hard, too, being in a group of them because you have to keep it confidential.

You can't go to their parent and say you know they're doing this and doing that, especially if you've already told them [your daughter and her friends] that you wouldn't. And there's one young lady who's just had really a difficult time this year. She's 13, she's got with the wrong group, quiet little girl, I mean hardly ever says anything, you could think she was the sweetest thang. She's cutting school, would be gone two or three days at a time, mom wouldn't know where she was. Come to find out she had this boyfriend that was much older. They were sexually active . . . [everything] just snowballed into a big huge thing and you know you look at yourself and think well okay, what went wrong, what was going on that she just went all into the left field, and I don't know the answer.

STRATEGISTS5: It's like they just be curious, they just wanna know . . .

Girls' choices of outfits and their influence on behavior constituted a great deal of concern by mothers. Several mothers indicated they routinely had fights with their daughters about what they wore. Indeed, they did not go into as much depth about the way in which television and advertising shape perceptions of girls, or about the types of marketing that are targeted specifically at girls. Rather, their concerns usually rested with other peer networks. The Revealers had an extended discussion about these issues.

REVEALERS1: For me, I would say someone who—it happens a lot to people who don't have stable homes; not all homes but a lot of times because they're out there looking for attention, you know, with a young man. And that's someone who's always switching from boyfriend to boyfriend, you know, who is with different partners. Because that does happen a lot and she tells me it happens a lot. But she's very aware and she's very mature for her age and she expresses herself really well. So, she's conscious of everything. She's talking to me and her father.

REVEALERS5: And I don't understand, I mean the way some of these girls dress, oh, my God!

[Agreement]

REVEALERS5: But then it's helpful when we make the clothes, too. I know with some of us, with our daughters being overweight, we have to make sure that we're in the—we want them to look young but we're forced to go to the older section. [Cross-talk, agreement, and discussion] Now, my daughter wears a size 11 and a 12 shoe. So, I'm trying to make sure that the heel is not too high and it's just, you know, trying to make sure that we pick out the clothes for them that makes them feel good about themselves too. So, that's a real issue.

REVEALERS2: Another real issue. Yeah.

REVEALERS5: But when I see these girls with short, short skirts on and I thought there was just certain things that we couldn't do when we—if you let them grow up too fast, they have nothing to look forward to.

[Someone says] Absolutely.

REVEALERS5: You know, occasionally I'll let me daughter get her nails done. But it has to be a special occasion. [agreement]. You have to work and you will pay for your own additional wants like . . . getting your eyebrows arched. Don't ask me for a Wii. Don't ask me to do anything that I work hard for that I consider a luxury right now.

[Agreement]

REVEALERS5: And when I see some of these girls out there that—

REVEALERS3: They've got everything. They get their nails done, their hair done, beads, everything.

REVEALERS5: You have to be 18, number one. And then you might get your nails done. But when they pop off, that's it!

This concern about dress from the mothers also relates to concerns about their daughters' physical development. Many mothers were aware of the public health claims that many African American girls were going into puberty faster than some of their white and Latina counterparts. As seen above in three focus groups, mothers also worried about how their daughters were dealing with sexual attention because they were "big" for their age and/or sexually developed. Styles of dress was an ongoing issue in their households and the subject of heated confrontations. In the Transitioners, one mother lamented that people tell her that her daughter is "big." In a moment of frustration, she turned to the others and said how much she does not like that others view her daughter as older and call her "big." She concluded by saying, "She's 13 and she's still a child."

In only one group did a mother challenge negative prevailing norms about girls and discuss the double standard of sexualized gender roles and expectations. A mother in the Strategists said her concern is less about labeling some girls as "bad girls." The bigger challenge, in her opinion, was helping girls find their way during the confusing time of adolescence. She found some agreement with that statement. They mostly thought it was media, peer pressure, and broken homes that contributed to certain kinds of behavior that they did not want their daughters emulating. As a whole, the mothers mostly downplayed hormones as helping to drive girls' experiences, which they did not do for boys and young men. Girls might be curious about sex, but they were not "driven" to have sex like boys. In the following exchange, the Strategists explored the negative consequences of double standards for men and women, while also remaining focused on pregnancy:

STRATEGISTS4: We gotta spend more time with 'em, because sometimes we let other things raise them almost, it's like you know, just because you're in the house with them, they may be in another room or whatever. But just like the Internet or the TV or whatever, just because they're in the house doesn't mean they're not getting that information.

STRATEGISTS2: I would like to talk about how society just views women and young girls . . . what comes to mind is the R. Kelly situation where everybody loves him. But then says, oh that bad girl, she was that, she was this, well what happened to him being responsible? Being an adult? Maybe she did come [to his room], but still to me that's inexcusable. I just get so mad, when people say oh it's the girl's fault. I mean people do it now, I hear people who have boys, boys for children saying oh these bad little girls and then they never want the boys to take any ownership and that just burns me up because it takes two! You can't put it all on the girl! And say oh well she went in willingly, okay, she offers, you don't have to take it! You know, stuff like that, so that.

STRATEGISTS5: It makes me mad how we as women always wind up on the short end of the stick. How we wind up pregnant and the guy goes away. It's like, okay, I got pregnant by myself and I took care by myself, but then he walks away, smelling like a rose. You don't have to see him ever again, but you will have that child for the rest of your life, you know? He'll pop up every once in a while if he choose to, he'll call if he wants to, you know. Or otherwise he can just act like you don't exist, to keep on goin', but then you're with that child, you know. And so it really bothers me . . . Why does it always happen to us that we get out there and we're supposed to love him and care about him but his idea of love and caring is not what not what we're thinking about, and then we wind up on the short end of the stick?

MODERATOR: Do we feel that we teach each other that because that has been taught to us by our mothers and we continue to put out there to our daughters and to our girls?

STRATEGISTS3: No, I think that we help them to adjust to the circumstances. Don't try to just sit around and blame . . . Just pick yourself up and address the situation and make the best of the situation, don't sit around and mope and complain about it. Do what you can, you a strong Black woman. Pull yourself up and take care of yourself, there's stuff out there we can do to better ourselves! And look at us, you know, rather than sit around and complain about being left alone, or the men that we used to love and don't love us and love somebody else, just pick yourself up and do what you got to do!

STRATEGISTS4: Well that's one thing that has to change. [Agreement]

STRATEGISTS3: It did change a lot!

STRATEGISTS4: They [men] can go sleep with a hundred women and people look at them like oh they're great and then if you see the woman, they say . . . they call her names, girls now, they all want more, they kinda, I don't know if they think guys are right because guys get away with it. They say, hey I can get away with it, too. I have the information so I can protect myself, and I'm a woman and I can do it all by myself. But you know you still have that cloud over your head.

STRATEGISTS3: And God forbid she wind up pregnant with children from every little different man. God forbid! God forbid! Look, look, God forbid she don't know who her baby's daddy is! God forbid! [Everyone laughs] Whew!

This group, while holding girls accountable for their actions, also acknowledged the double standards that structure much of social life for girls and women. The discussion of rapper R. Kelly is instructive, too, because Strategists2 names society's long-held excusal of rape and sexual assault by powerful men through victim-blaming and slut-shaming. She then makes the connection to these same gendered logics surrounding the R. Kelly controversy to what she hears people in her community say about young men (who may or may not be formally accused of rape or sexual assault). Strategists4 acknowledges that the terrain is different for young men and women and that young women openly seek to have more sexual agency and control in their lives. She, however, also acknowledges that while girls may want "more" and act on those desires, society's treatment and evaluation of girls has not radically shifted.

STDs

Like pregnancy, STDs allow mothers to reflect and compare their own adolescent experiences and interpret them through a comparative and nostalgic lens. Although the mothers collectively did not perceive HIV/AIDS as a major threat to their daughters' health, they were generally concerned about STDs. A few did think that STDs were a greater threat than pregnancy—though as I have argued above, their main concern by far was pregnancy. Many of the groups expressed the idea that kids generally have it harder now navigating sexual contact than they did when they were young women. Nostalgics begin our discussion and in this group they were generally not inclined to talk much about HIV/AIDS:

NOSTALGICS1: I have a couple friends who are teachers. And they were telling me that a high school teacher said that with the girls now, it's like, OK, to stay a virgin as the girls are doing oral sex because it's kind of like, you know, "All right. I'm a virgin. I can tell my mother I'm a virgin, yes. But meanwhile I'm here in the back giving head to this guy. And it's a good thing." And I mean it's OK, it's acceptable. And it's acceptable among the peers to do that. And so I heard that. So with my daughter, we've got to have a conversation. I ask her, "Is it sex if you are going down on a guy? Is that sex?" "Oh, mom!" she says. I say, "Is it sex? Yes, it is." She doesn't want to talk about it. But I'm like "It is sex and it's dangerous."

As the mothers reacted to her comment with murmurs and nods, she questioned the decision-making process of how some girls might think that certain sexual behaviors are OK. She exclaimed that STDs were a possibility and asked rhetorically why girls didn't know that. She concluded with:

So, it's just interesting, the change from when I was a kid. It was pregnancy was the issue. And now my greatest fear, even though I don't want the pregnancy, is to save her life. [Agreement] That, to me, is the ultimate issue.

A Strategist and a Transitioner echoed a similar observation:

STRATEGISTS4: I really want her to know that sex can kill, that literally sex can kill. So, that's my main thing that I worry about with her (when thinking about sex), with the STDs and the stuff that you can't get rid of.

TRANSITIONERS1: You know, that's why I try to teach my kids. And the reason why it concerns me, boys and little girls together, it concerns me about—the reason why I might get concerned about her health is because little boys whisper sweet nothings in your ear. And you [inaudible] and disgrace you and you end up "OK, my mama ain't gonna know it." [Agreement] And then you turn around and you do have— [cross-talk]. Condoms. You can talk about condoms [agreement]. They can talk them out of a condom. [Agreement] And then AIDS lies everywhere.

In the Strategists group, one of the mothers brought up HPV, the vaccine that protects against cervical cancer, and this sparked a discussion as well as an argument. There was some back and forth among the participants and, like the Nostalgics, they agreed that sex has higher consequences now:

STRATEGISTS6: Oh yeah, I've seen that on TV, I know I ain't gettin' none of that.

STRATEGISTS4: I went to a women's conference a couple of weeks ago and one of the mothers stood up and she said well, "What about the oral sex that all of them are having now, can you get HPV from that? and the speaker was like, "Yeah you can." And she also said what is so bad about that is that some people don't have any symptoms at all and so that's what I push. You can't look at somebody and tell if they're gonna get anything. And you may have it and not, you think that you are at a young age and you don't need to go to the doctor, you wait 'til you're 18 or 19 and you may not be able to have any kids by the time you go, it may have damaged you that much. So I would try to inform them that way because sometimes you know, you always hear that saying that what you don't know can't hurt you, yes it will. It can kill you.

STRATEGISTS5: Nowadays kids don't have sex, they have oral sex [talking over each other].

STRATEGISTS6: Yeah, that's what they been doing on the bus.

ALL: Yeah, on the bus, at school, in the bathrooms. [Multiple speakers]

The Nostalgics further compared and contrasted their experiences growing up as a sexual person in the past and now:

NOSTALGICS3: AIDS makes it really scary [agreement]. Think about it. And I mean it's hard growing up now. I wouldn't want to be a kid growing up now for anything. It's difficult.

NOSTALGICS2: I was in ninth grade in 1987 and sex education hadn't got to where it is now. We were putting condoms on bananas [laughs]. So, all of us knew. And you had to take that course. And my area still had some of the highest STD rates in the nation, OK? In the nation. And so, yeah, I don't play with that either. And, you know, it's very serious and I will talk to her about sex every single time, every single time; And, I'll say, "Not just this one thing, but it's these ten things could happen to you."

And some of those discussions have been really good for her as we go on. But that's—my biggest fear is about the lack of information that she's going to get under the abstinence policy. [Agreement] And knowing that I'm going to have to do that education myself. And I know a lot of people feel like that's the way it should be, right? But at the same time we're not responsible for vaccinating our children at home [agreement]. You know? What's worse, measles or AIDS? [Agreement] You know? I want every kid that my child goes to school with vaccinated!

. . . And it's not just a night of pleasure. You know, they're doing stuff in the bathroom stalls in school. They're doing stuff in the back of the bus. They're doing stuff everywhere.

Here we can note that not only is there general agreement about the threat of HIV/AIDS, in particular, but also that these mothers like the Strategists share a similar concern about where possible sexual activity for young people could occur.

The Experts were one of the few groups in which some mothers said that HIV was their daughters' biggest health risk. One mother elaborated about these fears and how she was proactive in getting her daughter to understand the risk.

EXPERTS2: If you're hanging out with a bunch of people who are let's go party, let's have sex all the time, then that invites other things into the door. In our church, they do a lot of HIV and AIDS seminars and I make her go and she's like, "Oh I don't want to go again." Yeah, come on, because you need to know this stuff . . . And then she won't be so gung ho to go out there and just settle for just anything.

So I really want her to be aware and I try to keep her busy and keep her focused and let her understand, whatever's going on with me I tell it. Because I want you to be able to go back and say, well when I was younger my mother handled it, so that's what works. That's what I feel is the biggest thing right now is just to be there.

Mothers' fears for their daughters are expressed through their concerns about pregnancy, the influence of other girls' behavior and cultural leniency, and to a lesser degree the possibility of their daughters contracting an STD. As I discuss below, these fears in many ways replicate the ideas that the mothers found difficult to navigate as young women. They also speak to the ways that these mothers feel that their ability to insulate their daughters from the changes in cultural norms (e.g., visibility and support of teenage mothers) is limited.

Conclusion

Upon examining the mothers' narratives, it is clear that mothers *are* communicating with daughters about sexual health and sexuality. This communication, however, is often fragmented, negative, or incomplete. Many mothers in the groups believe that they have broken with some of the confining norms that they experienced with their mothers when discussing sexuality and sexual health. These findings suggest, however, that some African American mothers may struggle with providing accurate and helpful sexual health information to their daughters despite their overall desire to do so. What emerges from questions about intimacy regarding their daughters is the way in which mothers also think about themselves and their choices. It reveals how single-parent and early-parent status may affect them in their perceptions of their daughters' needs and their communication styles. Additionally, many mothers have not had an opportunity to process their own possible regret or challenges about their own sexual history, which may contribute to them sending contradictory messages to their daughters about sexual intimacy.

This work makes a connection not just to the general challenging cultural context that African American women negotiate to become sexual beings, as other researchers have noted, but also how different regions as informed by memory and history potentially are shaping mothers' responses. Although not bound by the strictures of the Jim Crow South, the legacy of constrained economic and social challenges for African American women are still salient. They were raised by mothers who either did not have the tools to communicate effectively about sexual health or chose not to. Additionally, there continue to be strict and punishing norms for sexual behavior for young Black girls. As we saw in chapter 2, these mothers also face economic pressures and gendered realities in both the private and public spheres.

Mothers used a variety of communicative strategies in discussing sexuality with their daughters. Most used the direct method, which involved talking about sex often, and were opportunistic in when they could speak with their daughters (i.e., watching television, in the car, cooking, etc.). They observed their daughters with friends and then discussed issues or even searched rooms. They also used authority figures to confirm virginity. Single mothers and mothers who began having children at an early age seemed especially to rely on more invasive and confrontational strategies. This may be because they implicitly feel more worried about the social and economic implications of being an early mother, in particular.

Mothers are often using outdated "gendered" scripts that focus exclusively on daughters' virginity that do not take into account other potential high-risk sexual activities that their daughters may engage in. The mothers' messages may inhibit girls away from wanting to ask information not only about sex but also about how their bodies are changing and developing during puberty. A driving focus for many mothers are fears of an early pregnancy and perhaps an overvaluation of virginity. Given the national indicators about early sexual activity of young girls, this narrow focus for mothers on what counts as sex obscures the fact that their daughters may be engaging in sexual activity and are at risk for STDs. Other sexual behaviors that are not viewed as intercourse (from the mother's perspective) and therefore leave them "as a virgin" may contribute to daughters engaging in risky behavior (i.e., anal sex). In the focus groups with the daughters, we did not specifically ask about their sexual behaviors, but many of the daughters shared what their friends were doing, which included participating in a variety of sexual activities. Also, because mothers are so often focused on intercourse and virginity, they miss helping their daughters navigate a variety of feelings related to sexuality. This near uniformity of responses suggests the endurance of intergenerational sexual scripts that do not vary substantially across decades. Much of their concerns can be read as highly gendered, age-old, and crisis-dependent.

Another explanation for some of the communication gaps between mothers and daughters that this research uncovers might be that mothers who have had poor or troubled relationships with their daughters and/or have experienced early pregnancy or other early traumatic event during adolescence may have even greater trouble communicating effectively with their daughters about sexual health and intimacy. If this is true, then it may be useful for researchers to identify those dynamics earlier on when building interventions with mothers and daughters.

A major perceived derailer for their daughters' success is an early and unwanted pregnancy. Such a situation would create enormous pressures and challenges for their daughters. A few of the mothers disclosed that they had early pregnancies and had to cope with many adult realities quite early in life. That is often the motivation that drives their communicative styles. In the end, however, many of the mothers may not be very different than the mothers from whom they try to create a narrative distance.

The focus on teen pregnancy and also gendered peer pressure can be thought of as manifestations of respectability politics. Clothing and concern about other girls being more sexually advanced was a consistent theme in mothers' narratives. Clothing is a marker of status and ability to navigate social capital. Girls are often made responsible for managing sexual behavior through activities and presentation of self, which includes dress and behavior in public. Girls receive contradictory and inconsistent messages across different sectors of society about what is appropriate, and this is often mediated by region, race, ethnicity, and sexuality. The imposition of implicit respectability codes can have a more pernicious impact of sexual victimization and "slut-shaming."

Gendered peer pressure and respectability politics are interrelated and, I would argue, contribute in part to a silence in these narratives about pleasure and desire. As scholars have noted, pleasure and desire for Black women and girls is an understudied subject.[6] A few mothers expressed wanting their daughters to have a healthy sense of pleasure and desire. But overall, this was not a pressing concern, as reflected in the way in which the conversations about intimacy often moved quickly to talking about fears of the consequences of sex. There was little room for discovery (with either gender), sexual curiosity, and other sexual expression. This silence is undergirded by a focus on heterosexuality. The mothers were invested in affirming their daughters find appropriate male partners. Moreover, many mothers advocated abstaining from sexual contact until marriage and often held up marriage as an ideal for their daughters. Despite some of their own experiences that heterosexual living arrangements and/or marriage did not always bring themselves fulfillment, it is interesting to note how strongly this concept was expressed as an ideal. Although they were critical of negative male behavior, they tended to reinforce and accept it. They also implicitly accepted many norms of traditional male and female relationships. We might assume that some mothers in this group, from varying class backgrounds, may be more invested in marriage for their daughters, viewing it as an avenue for both social and economic capital. However, this seems less likely given the more uniform responses from mothers from across all income backgrounds.

Are there new scripts that can emerge over time that demonstrate the real material concerns about young Black girls but leave space for pleasure and desire? In discussing intimacy with the mothers, several groups acknowledged what would be helpful in their discussions with their daughters. Mothers expressed wanting and needing more resources to support themselves, cultivate additional communication skills, and see their daughters in new ways. They were interested in programs that would develop and/or deepen their daughters' self-esteem, confidence, and ability to navigate young womanhood. One mother offered that a holistically oriented program for girls "would be helpful because it gives the girls some other messages . . . not just don't have sex, you know, to boost their self-esteem and their sense of self-worth. I mean, really asking the question: Is the boy worthy? I mean really! Are you worthy of me? I mean I would love for my daughter to have that attitude."

We now turn to how the daughters' perceptions of sexuality and how they viewed their discussions of intimacy with their mothers.

5

"Mom, Can We Talk about Sex?"

Daughters and Sexuality

In the last chapter, we explored the ways in which mothers understood daughters' transition to womanhood and how they communicated about intimacy and sexuality. Most mothers felt connected to their daughters and were pleased with their level of communication. Overall, many mothers compared themselves to their own mothers and argued that they were not like them. Mothers in the focus groups believed that they were providing their daughters with a different and high-quality experience when it came to communicating about sexuality. This sense of distance from their mothers, their belief in their competence, interest, and commitment to communicating with their daughters, were cornerstones in mothers' narratives and a key feature in their identity as mothers. Their narratives, however, also revealed tensions about the quality of communication, the frequency and type of communication they had with their daughters. They ruminated about their own regrets and challenges, especially in the context of being either single mothers and/ or mothers who had their children at an early age.

This chapter turns to the daughters and explores how they wrestled with questions of intimacy and sexuality. As we saw in the health chapter, compared to the mothers, daughters did not always share their mothers' perceptions about the importance or value of health. Similarly, this chapter demonstrates the ways in which there is a mismatch for the majority of mothers in communicating with their daughters. Daughters characterize their mothers' communication with them as antagonistic, blaming, and challenging.

It is not universally true that these daughters could not talk to their mothers or did not receive sexual health information from them, but the majority expressed that they didn't approach their mothers for this kind of information. The majority of daughters did not feel that they could seek out information regarding sexual health from their mothers, and if they did, it was assumed by their mothers that they were already having sex. This gap in perception is striking given the mothers' narratives of openness, which is rarely mirrored in their daughters' language. For many, their mothers played an oppositional or antagonistic role because they talked about sexuality and relationships in ways that the daughters did not want to listen to and tried to avoid, or daughters felt like they could not talk with them at all.

The daughters' understanding of sex, intimacy, and relationships was an amalgamation of conversations with primary family members, friends, and media consumption. Daughters talked to friends, looked on the Internet, and took cues from the media as well as from other adult females. Sometimes fathers played an important role discussing sexuality. This pattern mirrors the way that the daughters approached their health. For many, mothers were to be avoided when it came to topics of sexuality.

Daughters felt like they had to navigate a range of intimacy choices by themselves. They had a hunger for knowledge about themselves and their bodies that was not met by their mothers, or most other adults. They perceived numerous silences about their mothers' intimate choices (e.g., timing of first sexual contact) and wanted to ask questions about the decisions that their mothers had made in the past (or were making in the present). For some, the silences around their mother's intimate choices created a barrier for daughters to raise questions about their own decision-making skills pertaining to their potential choices regarding relationships and intimacy.

In this chapter, I also demonstrate how girls make sense of and navigate these choices from a place of gendered expectations. Their narratives on the surface appear to be about mundane issues (i.e., fashion), but on further exploration reveal the ways in which ideas about gendered behavior shape and constrain their expectations and illuminate the micro-dynamics of gender.

We begin with how they define and understand sexuality.

Definitions and Perceptions

The girls ranged in thinking about sex, mostly in a traditional way (i.e., heterosexual intercourse), though they also spoke about oral sex (which for most of them did not count as sex since a girl could engage in that sexual act and could still refer to herself as virgin). Sometimes the girls defined sex as an emotional decision, an act, a type of behavior, or even a feeling. The Equalizers even suggested that the term itself might need rethinking:

EQUALIZERS1: People don't really use sex anymore, like the word. Boys don't. [Everyone talks over each other] females use that type of word, but boys are more like . . . [pauses]

MODERATOR: Blunt?

EQUALIZERS1: [laughs]

EQUALIZERS3: They be making up words sometimes just to describe [it].

EQUALIZERS1: Disrespectful words!

EQUALIZERS3: Yeah, they'll say stuff like "yeah I just got this girl last night" or "I beat that, yeah, I hit that" you know, or "I'm gone hit that" if a girl walks by.

EQUALIZERS1: I think to females it's more sacred, but to boys it's just like something . . . I feel like, like people put a lot on women, but not a lot on men about stuff, about sex and stuff. Like they're always like a female is a ho, but what about a boy? Why is he not a ho?

As noted in other chapters, the Equalizers had the most consistent focus on negative gender stereotypes. Further into the conversation, they picked up on another way that many members of the focus groups described sexuality as something sacred:

EQUALIZERS1: I feel like sex should be sacred, it should be something you do with someone special, like not just doing it with anyone just because they're there. I feel like it should be sacred.

Moderator directs a question to Equalizers1 and asks if she is talking about intercourse. Equalizers1 confirmed.

EQUALIZERS2: I agree with her. I mean, it's like the way you make life. And if that's not like sacred then what can we make sacred? Life is like the only thing that we have.

Most girls across the focus groups shared this idea that they wanted sex to be something special, important, and valued. Other descriptions of sex by the girls included "sex being a traumatic experience," and "sex is too casual by society's standards." In the case of the first reference, girls had talked to some friends that were sexually active and who did not have positive or pleasurable experiences.[1] Later in the chapter, when I discuss conversations that daughters would like to have with their mothers, the idea of sex as repeatedly painful and sometimes emotionally difficult is a salient one.

Although the Romantics talked clearly and in-depth about health, in much of their discussion around sexuality and intimacy, they used idealistic, sentimental, and metaphorical language. In comparison to the other groups, they honed in on romance and relationships. In this excerpt, they begin on a narrative path that will shape much of the rest of the conversation:

ROMANTICS1: My mother will sit down me with me and all of my friends and she'll tell us about everything, even if it makes us uncomfortable. [She'll talk about] like having like a simple like relationship to all the way to sex and child-birth and all that kind of stuff. She'll just sit us down and pull out some popcorn and some sodas. Like . . . "This is it. You can ask questions."

ROMANTICS2: My grandma sat me and my cousin down and explained an hour's worth of stuff, a lot of stuff.

MODERATOR: Stuff like what? Can you give me an example?

ROMANTICS2: Like sex and bad relationships and boys and keeping yourself healthy and not doing wrong things like smoking, getting pregnant too early. And my aunt sat us down again. Every time we go to her house, she sits us down or if she sees us talking to boys, she'll sit us down again.

Later in the conversation:

ROMANTICS2: My mom hasn't ever told me anything. My dad, he's told me about dates and stuff. But he hasn't really gotten to it. But my grandmother, she said always make sure that you find the key to your heart before you open the door. Ohhh! [Cross-talk and girls are animated]

ROMANTICS3: I like that.

ROMANTICS1: I like that!

[Agreement from other girls]

This comment about finding the key to your heart ignited the conversation for the girls. This was a metaphor for a decision to have sex with someone. They connected with this metaphor, and that became a focal point for much of the conversation. As it unfolded, they explored why people choose to have sex and what it meant to them. They defined having sex as "letting it go" and also "a one-night stand":

ROMANTICS1: Can I say something? Some people have sex 'cause they like how that person looks and some people may meet a person at the club and go home with them.

[Agreement]

ROMANTICS2: That's why I stick to that saying. Always find the key to your heart before you open the door.

[Agreement]

ROMANTICS1: To me it means intimacy and passion and relationships, with someone that you really care about.

ROMANTICS2: Not all the time—

ROMANTICS3: Not all the time with some people.

ROMANTICS2: [It means] Intercourse.

ROMANTICS3: A relationship—
ROMANTICS4: Mistakes.

Romantics3 mentioned that she had heard terrible things at school about sex from what other girls shared, and it scared her. Romantics4, who had not spoken much, said to Romantics2, "I like what you said about the heart," referencing the key metaphor again. There was some consensus in the group that this is perhaps the best way to make decisions about intimacy.

These exchanges reveal a few things: One is that mothers and other people are communicating with daughters about sexuality. Grandmothers also play a role in developing sexual norms. The Romantics, while solidly affirming their health and ability to talk with their mothers about health, were split on whether they could and would talk to their mothers about sexual topics. Their deliberations are further complicated by the fact that two girls began the conversation by stating that they could talk to their mothers about sexuality and intimacy but by the end of the conversation, reversed themselves and said that they could not. Despite this contradiction, the Romantics overall did not express the same level of tension about discussions with their mothers in comparison to the other focus groups.

The Equalizers perceived that talking about sex with adults, particularly parents, was taboo, yet in the following exchange, they conveyed that not talking about sex was unhelpful, as was the common adult refrain "Just don't do it." In this discussion, Equalizers4 recounts how she argued with her principal about a movie they were going to watch in school until someone discovered it contained a sex scene:

EQUALIZERS4: I was like why we can't watch it? It's just like sex and it should be, like—
EQUALIZERS3: —It's like a word that's forbidden from anybody sayin' it or doin' it.
EQUALIZERS4: I feel like people just don't talk about it enough so maybe that's why people don't know as much and people don't know the risk and all that kind of stuff.
EQUALIZERS3: A lot of girls just don't care. It's like now, like a lot of parents don't talk to their kids about it, they just like brush it off and be like okay I'm not talkin' about this.
EQUALIZERS4: Or they'll say just don't have sex and you can't tell, I'm sorry, you cannot tell a 14-year-old child, any teenager, you can't tell them don't have sex, they're gonna do the exact opposite. That's just something people our age do.
EQUALIZERS3: We don't listen to our parents, our parents will tell us don't go do this and you're like okay and [then] go do it.

Despite their criticisms about parents and speaking with them, Equalizers accorded school a high regard, valued teachers, and felt that teachers could act as confidants.

Across the groups, daughters' understanding of sex was that it was something that they should wait for, maybe not all the way until marriage, but until they were older. They found cues in their environment about waiting, as the Romantics indicate when they discussed a popular song:

ROMANTICS3: My mom, ever since she heard the new S.E.X. song by Lyfe Jennings, she's always saying, "Think before you let it go."

[Laughter] Ever since she heard that song, she's like "I like that! Think before you let it go. I like that." She keeps saying that. [Cross-talk] [Agreement]

ROMANTICS2: Yeah, I played it in my room one day, that song and I asked my mom to come and listen and I repeated the words, respect. [She sings a few lyrics.] She said, "Yeah, you better sing that kind of song."

The Moderator clarified that the girls were using the phrase "letting it go" as a way to talk about sex. They agreed that was what they were referring to. The girls discussed how sometimes music provided a good message that also aligned with what their mothers were telling them about not "giving it up." The Moderates also thought about sex overall as something to wait for. They, however, also intertwine the concept of waiting with religious beliefs and concepts:

MODERATES1: I'm pretty much grown so I know everything that I need to know.

MODERATES4: I don't exactly know everything because me and my mom don't talk seriously about sex, if we talk about it it's like a little joke. But like, I'm not a Christian, but I believe in God and I believe when people say you know wait 'til you're married to have intercourse. But my mom didn't wait or anything, so, what if something happens if I don't wait, or something like that, what if I get in trouble?

MODERATES5: Yeah, I'm a Christian, I'm actually a PK; I'm a preacher's kid. And I believe in God and at the same time I believe that you should wait until you're married. I personally believe that I'm not going to get married, so I don't know if I'm going to wait until I know that this is the right person and that I'm old enough and mature enough to handle a situation like that or if I'm going to just wait.

[MODERATES4 POSES THE QUESTION AGAIN: What if you meet someone before "it's the type of age for you to get married, and you wanna have that?"]

MODERATES5: I'm looking toward marriage, I'm just waiting until I'm emotionally ready and physically ready to deal with something like that because me personally, I don't have the time to think about all the consequences and repercussions and everything that goes along with it.

So far we have a window into how girls across the focus groups wrestled with the consistent theme that arose of waiting until marriage as an ideal. This connects to the ideals and messages that we saw mothers strongly express in chapter 4.

Waiting to be sexually active also poses its challenges. Below, the Moderates explored changes that take place from middle school to high school and the kinds of expectations and the pressures girls face:

MODERATOR: So when you have questions about stuff like that, about sex or about growing up or about being ready for different things, who do you ask those questions?

MODERATES2: I ask my sister.

MODERATES4: I don't ask questions because that doesn't come to my mind. Because anything I think about is just what I do and stuff like that, being my age, talking about boys and stuff, just being a pre-teen.

MODERATES3: When you're like, 10, 11, 12, and 13, and maybe until you are about 14 ½, it's just innocent, just talking about boys and how you [might] like him, but once you hit that 15, 16 mark, it's a whole new ball game.

MODERATES4: Really?

MODERATES5: What grade are you in?

MODERATES4: I'll be goin' into the seventh.

MODERATES2: It's just like once you start getting into middle school, you look around you . . . Hey everybody's talkin' about stuff that I don't really know about and should I know about this and—

MODERATES4: —it's kinda like you should learn, but it's like to a point where if you learn too much—

MODERATES5: [Everyone says] yeah, it's like you wanna know what people are talkin' about and should I know about this and is this right but you don't really know about it yet.

[Moderates3 repeats herself that "it's a whole new ball game" as a girl gets older. Others agree]

MODERATES3: Because then it's about the whole oral sex, because now what people are saying is oral sex isn't real sex because you can't get pregnant.

ALL: But it is!

MODERATES3: It is! If girls have sex they considered a ho, but if they have oral sex they still considered a ho . . .

MODERATES4: It's like what's the difference?

The girls mulled over the challenges around waiting to become sexually active, the slut-shaming of girls, and the possibility of contracting an STD:

MODERATES5: It's not even the name calling and all that, it's just that anything that I do that's gonna affect me in a big way like emotionally, that is considered a big thing to me whether it's oral or full intercourse. If it's gonna affect me in an emotional way on that big of a level then I consider it important.

MODERATES4: Yeah, 'cause like that friend that I had that's going to high school, she talks to me about that stuff because she knows and she has a boyfriend. She knows her limits and she wants to wait until she gets married too, and so when she talks to me about . . . yeah . . . [others say, it's okay!] it's like you know, what's the difference, she tells me, "Okay 'if you do this with somebody you can catch something regardless if it's sexual intercourse or anything else.

MODERATES3: And I think also with that and with the whole sex being general, sex is a really big emotional thing, it's really really emotional [said with emphasis]. While my aunt was pregnant with my cousin, no joke, my uncle left her. 'He was like oh, you got a baby, I don't wanna be with you, you know, it was just that one-night thing. And she got so distressed over that. I remember spending the night over with her and she was thinking about killing herself because he didn't want to be with her. That's a really big emotional thing when you have, that's like a connection you make with that person so really, I personally think wait 'til you get married 'til you know that connection's already there. And you know you know, you have waited and waited so you know that he ain't gonna leave you, or else he would have done it already. That's why I think wait until you get married.

MODERATES2: But, even if you wait 'til you get married, you can still catch a disease or something.

MODERATES3: Well, that too.

MODERATES1: Well, just the whole trust issue. Whether you trust somebody enough to believe that they're not going to go outside of the relationship. No matter what situation it is you still have a chance of getting something. But it's just like knowing your boundaries like right now like, majority of us we know how far we gonna go right now if we were with somebody and we know what we would do. But do you trust this person enough to think okay they're gonna stay with me after this or not?

Their conversation conveys a sentiment found across the other groups. Sex, besides the physical and emotional entanglements, also means negotiating social ideas about girls and socially appropriate behavior. It means figuring out one's boundaries. Some girls believe that they are not ready for that level of commitment and so therefore are wary. They also worry about a guy's commitment to them if they engage in sexual activity as well as possibly getting pregnant. Others like this girl from the Loners had been proactive; she went and talked to her health counselor at school and also researched STDs online:

LONERS2: I'm in a stage where I'm trying to make up my mind if I want to have sex, if that's something that I want to do because I really don't know. I really, I never had intercourse, but I'm trying to decide. You know, I want to 'cause some people make it sound good and some people make it sound dumb. And I'm kind of at that point where I'm researching certain things you can get. . . . Not a lot of people do that.

In all groups, concepts of sexuality, intimacy, and relationships were on the daughters' minds. They have been exposed through peer and popular culture about relationships, especially heterosexual ones. How girls defined and perceived sexuality and what they had learned about sexuality from others was primarily through a heterosexual frame. Homosexual and bisexual choices were not seen as valid for girls. In both the Experts and the Moderates groups, there was extensive conversation regarding homophobia, parents' thoughts about homosexuality as well as their own. Overall, the daughters were steeped in school culture and home life that could be defined as heterosexist and homophobic.

The Equalizers discussed rumors about sexuality. Two girls discussed how they go to schools that are labeled "bad" and also that there are "a lot of gays and lesbians":

EQUALIZERS1: I mean you can tell that there are some, but it's not like you hit the door, there they are all in the hallway and you just like he one, he one, he one, she one. I mean you can't point it out like that. There may be like ten, which you like walking through the hallway you see, but you're not gonna sit there and they're not gonna come up to you and be starin' at you. And people told my friend, they were gonna get hit on by a girl and stuff like that—

EQUALIZERS3: —What does that have to do with anything? Girls, I hate when people say like all gay girls wanna hit on you and stuff, it's not true.

EQUALIZERS1: Yeah, I got there, and if you make yourself known that that's not the way you roll, you cool with 'em, they're not gonna mess with you. I walked into school and I guess they just saw it that I'm not like that. Nobody's messed with me. So that definitely wasn't worth all that pressure. And I actually called my friends about it and was like where's the pressure 'cause it isn't as bad as y'all making it . . .

EQUALIZERS3: The year before I came people, the rumors were somebody got raped there and people were like yeah you need to be careful, don't be walkin' around Donaldson by yourself. I get to Donaldson I'm like what? Where are there people getting raped?

EQUALIZERS1: I mean they make it sound like every corner you turn and every little hallway there's something going on that indicates of what we talkin' about like what she said about people getting raped. It seems like every time you hit the corner there go a girl sitting there getting raped by some boy.

Equalizers3 confirmed that in her high school there was a rumor of lesbians raping straight girls. Equalizers1 argued that people exaggerate about how many gays and lesbians attend her school and also that the rumors that circulate about lesbians in her school are damaging. She indicated that many girls there believed the rumors and changed their behavior in going to the bathroom. She warned that people should not succumb to peer pressure. Also troubling in this exchange is Equalizers3's and Equalizers1's comments about sexual assault, especially about girls getting raped in school "by some boy." Neither participant elaborated on these comments and the moderator did not probe further, but the casual ease with which it was mentioned as a common occurrence is worrisome. Rumors shaped Equalizer1's perception of lesbian sexuality (and other LGBTQ students) and it minimized issues of sexual assault for both girls.

Among the Moderates there was a spirited discussion of how to reconcile one's personal religious beliefs with how to treat others that identify as LGBTQ individuals. Moderates1 said that after her mother saw two girls kiss in public, she had a strong and negative reaction, "She had a fit, she was like, 'If you ever do that and I catch you doing that you are out of my house, that's what she told me.' So I was just like, well, I don't have that thought in my mind but . . . okay, I know not to think it." After a lengthy back and forth exchange, one girl who had been relatively quiet and observant for most of the discussion about sexuality asked a question that had a high level of engagement among participants:

MODERATES1: I have a question, can I ask them something?

MODERATOR: Yes.

MODERATES1: Oh, I have a question like, Why do you think it's like a burden? Like to be gay? Why do you think it's a burden to the person that's gay?

MODERATES5: No! That's just like asking if it's a burden to be Black. It's just that everything that you are, there's always something about it that's gonna draw people to say something about you. That's, my personal opinion, I can't speak for anybody else or my father's ministry or anything like that, my personal beliefs is that if you choose to be gay, that's your lifestyle, I can't tell you whether it's right or wrong, I can only put my opinion in and if you choose that way then that's how you choose to live and of course there's always gonna be somebody that says, you're gonna go to hell for this and there's always gonna be somebody on the sidelines puttin' you down, but you can only live your life how you choose to live it and if that's how you choose to live then more power to you!

MODERATES1: So how do you feel about it?

MODERATES3: I agree with her that like that's your life, I can't tell you, don't be gay 'cause if you feel that way then you feel that way. But me personally, I have friends who are gay and I tend to get along with them better because I don't have to stress about saying this about a guy that I like, you know, saying it to another girl who likes the same guy . . . that kind of thing, but you know they're gay it's easier to talk to them about guys 'cause they [act] like girls. And gay guys are like the most fun to go shopping with.

There was some discussion between Moderates4 and Moderates5 as they wrestled with their religious convictions and feelings about having friends that identify as gay or lesbian:

MODERATES5: I mean I know that it's like confusing like you wanna speak to your beliefs, but at the same time you feel like they should be happy. But you have to decide how you're gonna mix your religious beliefs in with your life beliefs. Like, I believe in God and I believe that I don't personally think that homosexuality is right, but you have to have a tolerance because you can't just, you can't just put people down because they decide to do something, because that's their life you can't tell them how to live. So even though I might not personally agree with it, I'm not gonna put somebody down because they choose to do it, that's just like if she smokes, I'm not gonna be like oh, uh, you're just killing yourself, you're gonna die, and just sit here and tell her these things because I think she realizes the consequence and she knows what goes along with every situation she puts herself in, so I can't tell her how to live her life.

Moderates3 says she disagrees with her father, though that was what she was taught. She adds:

If they're gay, Black, white, Jew, whatever, it shouldn't matter as long as, if you love that person, love holds a standard by itself. So me telling somebody that you're going to hell because you're gay or you're not going to heaven because you're gay, it's not cool for me to say that because that's not me and I can't tell someone how to live they're life and I can't tell them that what they're doing is wrong, that they should change because of what I said. That's how I feel about it.

MODERATES2: Like when she said about your friend, you don't care if she's a lesbian. You're still her friend or whatever. Like with boys, they totally different.

ALL: Yeah.

MODERATES3: See, guys, they think the whole girl on girl thing is hot, but when it comes to guy on guy . . .

MODERATES2: They ready to kill.

MODERATES3: That and they isolate them.

MODERATES5: I actually think that if you're such a homophobe that you have to point it out every time you see it and you have to say something about it, then you're not secure in your own sexuality and there's some things in your own life that you need to look at. 'Cause that's their business. You do what you do as long as you're happy and you feel like you're in a secure relationship where you're not being emotionally or verbally abused or anything.

Everyone continued to stay engaged in the conversation as it slowly shifted to the concept of gendered behavior in dress and appearance. Moderates1 remained silent until she was asked if there was one thing that she wanted to tell her mother. That is when she disclosed that she identified as gay.

MODERATES1: Gosh, you put me on the spot! I really don't know like, like me and mom we really have like a weird kind of relationship because I'm really not as close to my mom like as you guys are. But like, I don't want her to worry about me because she gets worried about me all the time because I am gay. My mother says, "I don't want you to have to go through that, I don't want people to pick on you or talk about you or make fun of you." But, I just want her to know that I'm gonna be alright and that I'm dealing with it by myself and that, uh, I'm sorry [seems overwhelmed by emotion]. And I just want her to like not be worried about me so much, she's worried about me all the time, she's like people get hung, you know people get beat up being gay, so I don't want her to worry about me.

The discussion in both the Equalizers and Moderates is illustrative of concepts about sexuality that remain taboo within the daughters' worldview.

For many daughters in the focus group, sexuality and sexual orientation is defined by Judeo-Christian beliefs and values. These can present challenges for girls who identify as bisexual or gay or other sexual identities on the LGBTQ spectrum as they may have fewer support systems to help them navigate developing a sense of self and/or healthy relationships. Narrowly defined concepts of sexuality can also negatively impact heterosexual girls' experiences as they find themselves in friendship, work, and social circles with LGBTQ people.[2]

Communicating with Mothers

The groups ranged widely in the kinds of conversations they had with mothers and other figures about sex. In the Distrusters group, several other people besides mothers were mentioned as having talked about sexuality, intimacy, and relationships.

MODERATOR: So, what has your mother shared with you about intimacy or being close to somebody? Have you heard a conversation?

DISTRUSTERS1: I've had the boyfriend conversation, but that's it.

MODERATOR: What do you mean, you had a "boyfriend conversation"?

DISTRUSTERS1: Well, my dad is crazy. We talk about everything. My dad, he was talking about that I've got to watch myself if I do have a boyfriend because you don't know when a boy might use you. So, you have to look out for signs. So he says, "Wait to find that person is the one for you." Because if not, it's not even gonna work out. You're gonna get like a divorce in like five seconds.

DISTRUSTERS2: I had a conversation with my sister. And she said you should not cheat on them [boyfriends], but just have your one dude on the side [as a friend], you know, to talk to just in case your boyfriend breaks up with you.

DISTRUSTERS1: I agree on that. Your man or your boyfriend or your husband might not tell you everything that's in the handbooks about men. So, you have that person that will tell you everything.

This elicited a spirited conversation about "friends on the side" that, from the girls' perspective, are another way to access resources and find out about guys without necessarily having a sexual relationship.

As illustrated in the example above, fathers also play a role in shaping girls' perceptions of sex. Fathers' communication about sexuality sometimes resembled mothers' admonitions about boys, other times, daughters experienced a sharp contrast between the ease with which fathers engaged their brothers about sexuality, compared to them:

EQUALIZERS3: It's like, at my household, my dad will talk to my brother all day long about having sex and stuff like that, but when it comes to me, my mom, my dad, as soon as I say like dad do you want to talk about it with me, he's like oh, where's your mother.

EQUALIZERS1: Yeah, thank you.

EQUALIZERS3: He'll just like call mom and she'll come in there and she'll be like what's the problem and he'll tell her and stuff like that. He treats the two of us different, it's like we live in like two different households and it's like in a lot of people's minds, like it's okay for a boy to go out there and get any girl, but when it comes down to my daughter you can't touch her. So . . .

There is continued discussion—and a lot of agreement—about how fathers treat their daughters and sons differently. We will revisit their sense of injustice and double standards later in the chapter.

"I Learned It All on My Own"

While the mothers often presented a unified narrative of openness and inclusion about intimacy and sexuality in talking to their daughters, this narrative was not affirmed by the daughters' discussions. Despite the mothers' expressed interest in communicating about sexuality and intimacy, the majority of the daughters indicated that they did not or would not turn to their mothers for advice related to sexuality and/or sexual health. They spoke primarily with their sisters, female friends, and aunts about sex and intimacy. They also often consulted the Internet to seek answers to their questions. Some daughters spoke with their mothers about sex, but the majority felt those conversations were confrontational, authoritative, and accusatory. The majority of the daughters did not feel they could have an open conversation with their mother about sex.

When their mothers spoke with them about sex, they told them to "wait until they were married" or "in a committed relationship"; "to be safe" (use a condom) or "cautious." They stressed messages that presented sex as something that can have negative consequences for their daughters' futures. Moreover, I found that daughters suggested that they often were not quite sure *what* their mother was trying to convey when discussing topics of sex and sexuality. These are quotes from different speakers from three different focus groups that highlight some of the ways daughters discussed their communication with their mothers:

- "No, my mom just told me to wait. She's like wait until you're ready or she said if I had it my way you should wait 'til you're married, but she just said wait until you're ready and you feel that the time is right."
- "If you're really gonna have sex at this age, then have protection."
- "When I got my—well, when my period started, my mama, she just said, "we don't need to have a talk about it. You already know the deal." [Laughter] [Two quotes above are from the same group]
- "I mean because everything that I have learned so far [about relationships and sex], I have had to learn on my own."
- "My mom never really talked to me about sex. I learned it all on my own."
- "My mom hasn't ever told me anything. My dad, he's told me about dates and stuff. But he hasn't really gotten into it."
- "My mom used to say, "not until you're married." Now she just says [wait] a little while before you get married. I'm like, I guess that's the same thing."

Daughters presented a consistent narrative that if they were curious about sex, sexuality, and even relationships, they had to take the initiative and "learn on their own." This placed daughters in a position where they felt it was up to them to go out and seek information.

One striking example of this comes from the Equalizers, who were daughters of the Experts group, which ranked very highly in being open and included a medical doctor and health educators. Here is a snippet from their discussion in which they had been asked to recall what their mothers shared with them about intimacy. The discussion begins with an unusually long pause for this group who had up until this moment been talking consistently fast:

EQUALIZERS4: Absolutely nothing.
MODERATOR: Nothing?
　　One participant asks for clarification, "Are you talking about relationships and stuff like that?"
MODERATOR: Everything.
EQUALIZERS3: Uh, I don't know, my mom just tells me to like, I don't, we don't really talk about. Well, we do talk about my relationships, but not really. She's not gonna tell me anything.
MODERATOR: So when you do have those conversations, what are those conversations about?

EQUALIZERS3: She asks me about how he treats me, does he ask me my opinion on things, when are we gonna, you know, have sex, or stuff like that.

. . .

EQUALIZERS2: For some reason she doesn't really talk to me that much about this stuff, she only talks to my sister about it. I don't know, so when she tells my sister . . . my sister and I are really close, she's four years older than me. And she comes back and tells me stuff that my mom told her about when my mom was younger and for some reason my mom just won't tell me. So I mean, I guess my sister and my mom sort of work together to do this stuff.

The moderator asks if there are others in their lives that they talk to about these issues.

EQUALIZERS3: My aunt.
EQUALIZERS 4: My sister.
MODERATOR: Your sister? And your aunt? And describe those conversations. What do you talk about specifically?
EQUALIZERS4: She asks me questions about me and my relationships and am I alright and you know, things like that.
EQUALIZERS1: I'm kind of close with my mom because we're so, our ages are so close together, so I'm really close to my mom, we talk about that kind of stuff.
MODERATOR: Would the rest of you feel the same way or is it different for your situation?
EQUALIZERS3: I'm not really close to her (my mother), I'm close to her, but we don't talk about stuff like that. I'm not really home to talk to her, I'm always at my aunt's house, so that's why I have the time to talk to her [aunt].

There was some back and forth here—two of the several girls said that they were close to their mothers, but they did not talk much about sex and intimacy.

In the Loners group, we see some similar patterns of discussion when compared to the Equalizers. Though in this group there is no pause or uncomfortable silence—one of the participants spoke up:

LONERS1: Of course. [Laughter] OK. My mom, she tells me stuff. One thing that I hate that she says to me is "don't have sex." It drives me to the brink. [Cross-talk]
MODERATOR: Why do you hate that?
LONERS1: This is why I hate that, because if somebody—and this is just for anything—if somebody keeps telling me not to do something, I tend to be like

"oh, so, it must be good if you're keeping something away from me. Or are you telling me that I'm not going to do it like I'm your slave. I understand that you're my mother but you still have to treat me with some respect because you want respect back. And when she tells me "don't have sex," I feel like "oh, so it must be good if you're trying to keep"—you know what I'm saying? Or it could be bad. But it doesn't really matter. She could keep telling me not to do something. But I feel like, out of no disrespect to anybody, but I feel like no matter what they tell you, you are your own person and you make your own decisions . . . I tell the truth. I'm sorry. I cannot lie. I say, you know, "part of being a parent is being a guide to your child. And I appreciate that. But also you have to realize that sooner or later I'm gonna grow up and I'm going to be an adult. And, you know, you're not going to always be there for me. You can give me guidance, but don't push your problems or what you want me to do onto me. You can tell me what you think might be best for me. But don't tell me what I am and I ain't gonna do 'cause I'm still gonna do what I want to do." And that's just being true.

Loner1 keeps talking with intensity. Others in the group nod and agree.

LONERS1: If I want to have sex, I'm gonna have sex. If I don't, I'm not. That's just how I feel about it. I'm not gonna say it's good or bad because I wouldn't teach my children that it was bad. I wouldn't want them to lie to me and when my mom tells me "you're not gonna do it," it makes me feel like I can't come to her and talk to her about anything. It kind of pushes me away because she won't ask me why I did it. She won't even sit down and talk to me about it. She just says, "You're not going to do it and that's the end of it!" So, everything I learned about sex, I learned from somebody else; I learned it from somebody else because I couldn't go to her for that.
[Emphatically delivered]

This is one of the few instances in which one of the girls disclosed that she is sexually active. Girls present a consistent narrative of having to take charge of learning about their bodies and sexuality. And despite their mothers' active engagement, that engagement did not translate to daughters feeling safe enough to talk with them.

This lack of discussion about sex and sexuality was frequently contrasted with stories about the sexual information and encouragement that was provided to their male siblings (both older and younger) from their mothers and fathers. Daughters discussed the effort to seek out information and, in some cases, even hid relationships with others in contrast with their male siblings. Participants discussed that male siblings were allowed more freedom to date and openly pursue sexual activity. Daughters noticed the role of double standards operating about the expectations of sexual behavior for them versus other male members in their household, like brothers. Daughters were keenly aware that their brothers were governed by different rules about sexual behavior than they were. They expressed frustration and confusion at this treatment. These narratives arose prominently in three of the five focus groups. One participant from the Equalizers described a common experience for many of the girls in the focus groups:

EQUALIZERS2: And then I want to ask her like why she isn't telling me, or why she doesn't like think to talk to me about this stuff [about sex]. Like when, so my brothers have like their girlfriends over all the time and like I have a few guy friends over with a lot of my other girlfriends we're back watching a movie and then my mom like calls me out of the room and takes me to the kitchen and asks me to keep the door open and then lets me go back. And then like the next morning my brother and his girlfriend like come down out of his room together and she sits down and eat breakfast with us and my parents don't act like it's strange at all.

After identifying a double standard, the girls homed in on how it manifests:

EQUALIZERS1: I feel the same way. My father's more of like the, the more open type you know. My brother does a lot of stuff, but I don't live with my father so you know, but when it comes to like my little sisters and me, it's like you know, no boy's gonna touch her, or when I was younger, my dad used to be really like overprotective. He's a huge man, he's like yah! He would like walk up there and take a guy! So it's like, don't you touch my daughters, but you know my brother he'll go over there and drop him over at his little girlfriend's house and he's the only boy there!
EQUALIZERS3: Yeah it's like the parents, like dads, they just think that girls are supposed to sit right there in their back pocket and not move and nobody's supposed to come up to 'em, but they don't really think that the person that they son is messing with is somebody else's daughter.

The Loners' perceptions about their treatment versus their brothers' arose when we asked the question, "What is one thing that you would share if you could share with your mom about your feelings in becoming a young woman." Loners3 and Loners4 offer their observations about their brothers and the different treatment received. There is a lot of cross-talk and agreement from the other participants.

LONERS3: I have a younger brother and for some reason my mama treats us completely different because I'm a girl and he's a boy and he gets to do a whole lot of stuff that I can't do and I'm older. My brother is very, very immature, like very. [Cross-talk] He acts like a baby. My mama still treats him like a baby. He acts like that.

She goes on and makes general comments about her brother that sound light-hearted, but then her demeanor changed:

And I don't understand but when I talk to my mama about it, I don't think she—I think she's in denial of that. He ain't right. [Laughter] But she feels completely different on issues about curfews or dating and stuff like that. It's because I'm not a boy, I can't do nothing of the stuff that she allows him to do. It really bothers me. And I don't think that's fair. And I tell her all the time, "I'm not going to do this to my little girl when I have one" and she's like "I said the same things when I was your age when my mom used to make me do stuff." But I think I'm actually gonna be completely different because I think that's just unfair. It is completely unfair.

LONERS4: I don't understand that either because, like, my brother, when he was ten he could have a girlfriend. And she used to could come over to the house and stuff. And I'm 15 and she says I have to wait till I'm 16. And I'm like, "Come on, now! That's six years. Ten and sixteen." I mean—and she's like "Well, he's a boy and boys are different." And I'm like "How are they different? They are the ones who want to have sex and like Come on, let's have sex." I would be the one who's like "No, I'm not ready for that yet." So, I don't understand why she's like "You're a girl." Like that don't make no sense to me. I'm 16. I'm old enough to have a boyfriend. I can't even talk on the phone to boys. And I'm like, "He had a girlfriend at ten and I can't talk to a boy?" I don't understand. Like I wish I could talk to her. But if I said something, she'd say like I'm grown or something like that. Like she'll say something stupid. [All delivered emphatically]

Before moving to the next theme, it is important to note that in contrast to sexual discussions with mothers that daughters perceived as stressing what "not to do," there were rare comments from daughters that suggested they had open, accurate, and positive conversations about sexual health. Below is one that stands out from the Romantics:

My mother says make sure you have a condom, make sure that you are perfectly OK with it and make sure that if you say "no," that he understands what "no" is. Make sure that you know the consequences of it, that there is a chance that you could get pregnant and that you're ready to take that on. Oh, she says to take a test, get an HIV test. Even if you know you don't have it, just get it anyway and make sure he gets it too. Make sure you see the little paper. And, oh, she says make sure it's not in her house. [Laughter from her and other girls]

This comment was striking in that it was one of the few positive comments made by daughters that convey several interlinked ideas. In this we see the mother conveying the importance of making decisions regarding sexuality, the importance for a young woman to not feel coerced into sexual activity, and also an explicit concern about STDs, including HIV/AIDS. We also can note that in this instance, the daughter is assumed to be able to discern how a young man may handle being told no in a sexual situation prior to being in that situation. We can also note that in this communication between mother and daughter, the language of pleasure is seemingly absent.

"There Are So Many Things I Want to Know"

Daughters are rarely asked what they would like to know from mother figures regarding relationships, intimacy, and sexual behavior. There were two areas that daughters in our focus groups identified as topics of conversation they would like to explore with mother figures. These included sexual health basics and how to handle situations that might lead to a more serious or intimate relationship.

Daughters wanted to know more about how their bodies worked as they moved into puberty, or if they were already in puberty then they wanted to know about sexual health basics. This included questions like "can one get pregnant if they have sex during their period?" to "does it hurt when you have sex?" They also wanted to know about sexual education and HIV/AIDS. They often had to seek out this information from other caregivers, friends, or the Internet. They frequently asked the focus group moderators basic sexual health questions. They wanted less of the narrative about "what not to do" and more about what they could do in relationships if they felt comfortable with a person. Daughters often wanted to probe their mothers' choices and past experiences in relationships. The daughters frequently picked up on regret or confusion about their mothers' choices. This seemed to be especially true if they knew their mother had experienced an early and/or unplanned pregnancy. This makes us wonder about the ways in which mothers indirectly communicate some of their choices regarding intimacy and how daughters perceive them.

They wanted help with complex decision-making skills related to interactions with boys. For example, one girl asked, "What if you are at a party or whatnot and all of a sudden this boy you've known and liked wants to change to another level? What do you do?" More broadly, I would argue that the girls were trying to make sense of the formal and informal rules that govern gendered behavior in relation to everything from self-presentation to dating. They wondered aloud about how boys are not penalized for dating many girls (sometimes dating more than one girl at the same time), or expressing desire for sex and enjoying being active, sexual beings. They also described situations where boys they knew had gotten a girl pregnant but did not seem to face the same social consequences as the pregnant girls themselves. The daughters did not seem to be able to place themselves in a narrative that easily affirmed sexuality or sexual interest.

One of the ways that the girls made sense of gendered messages was to rely on the model of "good girls," and "bad girls" or "hos," a typical schema available to young women and reinforced through daily cultural interactions with peers, parents, television, music, movies, and popular culture generally. Good girls are those that follow the gendered rules and do not express sexual interest (or if so, in a coded way), bad girls and hos are ones that attract and engage male attention. This exchange between the Equalizers illustrates several aspects of this topic. Equalizers3 tells the group that she feels pressure from her family to do well in school:

EQUALIZERS4: [Agrees generally] A lot of girls put a stereotype on girls, so a lot of boys look at you as like you ain't nothing but another ho. I mean I'm not a ho, but people put that out there, people say you all are in that same stereotype. So some of my friends do act like that then . . . Even if I go to the mall with my friends, we have people look us up and down and stuff like that. I may not even go to the mall with my friends that do act fast and stuff like that, but I mean—

EQUALIZERS1: —They'll do that anyways, guys'll look you up and down like you got something—

EQUALIZERS4: —But I'm talking about grown women and stuff like that.

EQUALIZERS1: Yeah, that's just rude, I hate that mess.

EQUALIZERS3: I feel like I'm always pressured to fight with somebody.

EQUALIZERS1: Yeah! Like it feels like girls are just pushing me sometimes.

EQUALIZERS3: They do stuff just because they know it's going to irritate you. They'll look you up and down.

EQUALIZERS1: Or look at your boyfriend and he's standing right there by you!

EQUALIZERS3: I had one girl come up to me (she's in the same class as me) with her friends like I'm going to get her man, I'm going to get her man. So next thing I know she's out there flirting with him. I mean boys they don't have common sense so of course they are going to flirt back, so he was flirting back with her—

EQUALIZERS4: —Not all boys—

EQUALIZERS3: Okay not all boys but some boys, they do flirt back. And so, it really does feel like you're being pressured to fight.

In this exchange we can observe a few things. Equalizers1 indicated that she wanted to distance herself from girls labeled "fast." The term fast is a common colloquialism, especially in African American culture that connotes sexual promiscuity or acting in ways that are inconsistent with being a young girl or respectable woman. The term can also mean possessing knowledge befitting a grown woman. What is interesting is the rebuttal by Equalizers4 that suggests even if one does not associate with girls labeled in that way, they will still be governed by masculinist ideas of power and control. This passage also informs us of how girls are beginning to understand that they participate in a culture that encourages them to be on display for young men. Their larger observation about boys and masculine behavior slips away from the participants and they returned to the easier target of other girls. The entanglements that ensued became structured around negotiating young male desire and competition.

The Distrusters were also full of questions. In this group there was some back and forth as they worked through a question posed by Distrusters1:

DISTRUSTERS1: I have one. Why just hook up? Why don't they want to have a full-time relationship? That's what I want to know.

This was echoed by one other girl and then was answered by another participant:

DISTRUSTERS3: You know, you are friends and you just hook up, real cool. Whenever the girl wants to do it [have sex], they just call each other. That's what it is.

DISTRUSTERS1: How come boys don't just take the responsibility? If you know you slept with that girl, be a man and tell her that, OK, this might be or this might not be my child. Be a man and just come out and tell. Don't be like "oh, it's not my child" or you think you're going to get a reputation of being a slut or whatever. No. Be a man and do what you've got to do.

This conversation led to a debate among the girls as to why some people avoid telling a potential sexual partner that they are HIV-positive.

In this exchange, the Loners echoed observations from girls in other groups about some of the consequences of asking certain kinds questions of their mothers:

LONERS1: I wanted to ask her something, but if I ask her she would probably think that I was about to go have sex. One time I asked her like could you get pregnant if you had sex in the pool. And then she was like "Well, you went to the pool today." What? [Laughter] I was like "No!" And then I wanted to ask her about, you know how people talk about when you first do it, like it's supposed to hurt or whatever. I wanted to ask her because I was thinking about doing it or whatever. But I didn't want her to know. I just wanted to see what she was going to say. But I didn't ever ask her because I knew she would be like "Now, you can't go to this party because you'll probably decide to have sex."

[One time I told] my mom about how my friend had got pregnant. She had unprotected sex. My mom was like "Oh, you can't hang out with her, you might be doing it." I told her honestly if I was going to do something like that, I wouldn't tell you because you're not gonna change my opinion."

[Cross-talk about various questions. Loners1 talks about not sugarcoating sensitive issues because it doesn't earn you respect.]

LONERS1: Yeah, but you can't ask your parents that. I don't feel like I can ask mama that because then they'll be wondering. I think if you ask them questions about sex they'll think that you want to go have it. They don't just think "oh, they just want to know." They're thinking "oh, she must want to go have sex when she's asking these questions." That's what I think.

Before the moderator has time to respond, another girl jumps in:

LONERS3: Can I ask you a question about that? I don't understand why parents don't—they don't think about stuff like the way we do. OK, if you don't talk to your child about certain things, especially stuff like sex or drugs, if you do not talk to your child, then they got to go get information from somewhere else, nine times out of ten they will go and they will do it just because they don't feel open to go talk to their parents about stuff. And that's how I feel now. I feel like "OK, well, if you can't talk to me about it, I'll find out from somebody else." When I find out from somebody else, it's like one of my peers and they're telling you "oh, it's good!"
[Agreement]

Some of their interests took on particularly difficult or challenging things for them to understand, as addressed by the Equalizers:

EQUALIZERS1: My mom had me when she was 14, so I've always wanted to ask my mom like why didn't you get an abortion. People told her you should get an abortion 'cause you're 14 years old and you're not gonna make it anywhere and all kinds a stuff. And I just wanted to ask my mom like why didn't you get one, like what made you not get one, because she told me at one point she was close to getting one. I've always wanted to ask her that, but I thought that might hurt her feelings a little bit to ask her something like that.

EQUALIZERS4: I mean I can't ask mom that 'cause she had me when she was 21, but she did have my brother when she was young and my brother does ask her questions like that and she said, once you are carrying a child for such a long time, you start to get attached to it. But I mean, there's nothing really that I'd ask my mom, because I'm the middle child so my mom tells me about everything. Every mistake she made with my brother, she doesn't want to make that mistake again. And I have a little sister so, she says you know whatever mistakes I made with you I don't want to make the same mistakes with her. So, she just, she says I wanna have an open relationship so we talk about everything.

The daughters' questions were numerous and wide-ranging, and they spanned across the groups. Girls would go out in pursuit of this knowledge, sometimes asking older siblings and friends, occasionally asking other adults, but most often they turned to the Internet and popular culture. Their mothers might be surprised at the depth and kinds of questions their daughters wanted to ask them.

What Would You Tell Your Friend? Navigating "Good" Girl and "Bad" Girl Culture

How do girls navigate their position as "respectable" and "good girls," a gendered and racialized formation? What are the pressures they face and how do they discuss other girls' roles as well as their own in this complex dance? How do they express disapproval of one another and how does that demonstrate internalized gender norms? One of the salient themes in comprehending how daughters understand their sexuality and communication about it is how they think about their own and other, similarly aged girls' behavior. Their perceptions provide a window into understanding the context of their decision making. Through this lens we see the tensions, contradictions, and warning signs accompanying these daughters' journeys into womanhood.

In the focus groups, we posed a scenario to the daughters for discussion. Scenarios are a useful tool in focus groups, especially in working with children and adolescents.[3] Scenarios and other participatory exercises allow researchers to understand how respondents think about an issue, particularly one that might be socially embarrassing or stigmatizing, but do not put respondents on the spot as the scenario is divorced from themselves. The scenario asked them to respond to their friend who had been asked to come to a Halloween party dressed as a "ho" by their boyfriend, who was going to be dressed as a pimp.[4] The scenario was offered later in the session after the group had been talking for some time and rapport was established. This scenario revealed their conceptualizations about sexuality, behavior, and dress that were hinted at previously throughout most of the interview.

The scenario discussions highlight the very real-world challenges many girls already faced and were navigating. In discussing the scenario there was consensus in the majority of groups that this could happen in real life. It resonated with them. They acknowledged that girls feel pressure to conform to male standards of "how to look like a girl" because representations of sexuality across popular culture, especially music videos. They also indicated that they knew of situations when girls *had* been asked by boys to dress in ways that both the participants and their friends found uncomfortable. They knew some boys who had said to their girlfriends, "I'm your pimp." In their world, they were already exposed to situations where boys wanted to act out fantasies that, according to the participants, tended to disadvantage the girl involved. They also cited rap and hip-hop videos that many boys they knew had viewed and how these boys often suggested to them and their friends that they could dress like the models and "video babes."

Across all the groups, the majority of girls said that they thought that their friend was ill-advised and misguided to do such a thing, and they said that they would stress for her not to do it. In responding to this scenario, girls discussed talking to their friend in a kind way and being supportive. One daughter in the Romantics said, "I'm going to stick by you if it goes downhill from there." Others said similar things along the lines of, "I would sit down and talk to them." A creative response was offered by one girl in the Distrusters group, who claimed she would reverse the tables by saying, "I'd be the pimp and make him dress like the ho."

In some groups they also offered several reasons why a girl *might* agree to dress in a way that made her feel uncomfortable, including: she had been previously sexually abused, she had no parental figures, and she possessed very low self-esteem. During the scenario discussion, daughters talked about self-esteem and how popular culture can devalue girls. One of the Equalizers, a group that was concerned with gendered treatment, made a connection between media, racialized gendered relations, and their impact on girls:

> I mean, actually me, I would ask her, you know, if she was my friend I would ask her why would she want to portray herself like that, you know? Because she should have enough self-respect for herself not to even play with something like that even if it was a joke. I take stuff like that seriously because the way that the media portrays women, African American males, or any type of male for that matter [are portrayed as] looking down on females now. "Oh, that's my ho." "Oh, I cheated on her." "Oh, I did this. Oh, I did that." I wouldn't even put myself in that situation so anybody could look at me like that.

Some of the girls admitted that dressing as a "ho" was possible or even allowable because traditional rules about dress and behavior were often broken during Halloween. Most groups conveyed that there would be negative consequences for the girl if she decided to undertake such an action. They said that the girl was likely to be stigmatized and shamed by other girls and boys at the party.

Below we draw on the Equalizers and Moderates discussions, as they were lengthy, animated, and similar in tone to the other groups. The Equalizers began the discussion with the kinds of gendered dynamics that they encountered in school and in which they saw their friends participate:

EQUALIZERS4: My mom doesn't like for me to say yeah, I'm a pimp, you know how people say, oh I'm a pimp.

EQUALIZERS3: My mom hates those songs.

EQUALIZERS4: My mama doesn't like that (either) because a ho is a person that gets beat by a pimp, he takes all her money, she's like nothing, rapes her, let men, you know she does oral sex on men for money, but she doesn't get any of the money. So my mama always tells me stuff like that, so I would tell my friend you know, don't do that, you should respect yourself enough to not dress as a ho, because your boyfriend does not pimp you. You're not going outside and having sex with people or having oral sex for money.

So why would you do that? Why would you pretend to be . . . ? I think people think that's cute to be a pimp and a ho, people think that's cute—

EQUALIZERS3: I mean like in school, a lot of boys say that, they'll be like, "Oh I'm her pimp and stuff like that—"

EQUALIZERS4: Talking about prostitutes—

EQUALIZERS3: Yeah, it's like boys that have a lot of groupies. It's like boys that have a lot of girls that are always around them. They're like yeah, these my hos right here. And I mean, you [the girl] is in the gutter and they're smiling. And I'm like that's not cute, that's not a cute thing to go off of. If he puts you out there like that then there's a problem, it means he really doesn't care about you. But, if they want to be that way, I mean you can't save the world, but you can save a friend.

EQUALIZERS1: If her boyfriend really cared about her, he would say I don't think that's a smart thing for us to be for Halloween. I mean if he really cared about her then he would tell everybody, I'm not sure about those costumes. . . . One year, I wasn't a ho, but I was a hoochie [at a party]. Just to be different . . . I went wearing a wig with my nails done and stuff.

EQUALIZERS2: I mean the boyfriend really should have thought about it because does he really want a bunch of other guys coming up to his girlfriend and being like all over her? If my boyfriend wore something that made like a bunch of girls like flock around him and be like all over him I'd be mad, I'd be like go away, he's my boyfriend! [All laugh]

EQUALIZERS1: Thank you!

EQUALIZERS2: I just think it's stupid, it's an all-around stupid idea, why would you want to do it?

Equalizer1 indicated she had a friend whose boyfriend had multiple girlfriends. She reiterated that the friend thought it was "cute." Her tone was dismissive.

She was like that's alright, that's alright, I'm his main one! And I'm like but he done told the other three girls the same thing and I mean like they think that was cute, they was goin' around school and all three of 'em were on him and everything and . . . I was just like that is just nasty.

EQUALIZERS3: That look like a pimp right there, that's how a pimp, I'm sorry I'm not tryin' to call your friend a ho or nothing, I'm sorry, but she made herself look like a ho right there, because he walkin' around with three women, that's what people expect for a . . . Have you ever realized when a boy is around a group of girls it's like, 'Oh, I'm a pimp?'

EQUALIZERS1: I actually did tell her that was what she looked like. She does put herself out there. As a friend, in certain situations, it is your duty to tell the truth. To be like hey, you's a ho, so you might want to calm that down.

MODERATOR: What did she say in response?

EQUALIZERS1: She gets mad. She says, "You're not supposed to say that to me." So, I've only told her once—that one time.

EQUALIZERS4: See I have a friend that tells me like she's nasty, she's just nasty, just nasty. She's like made comments like once I'm a ho I can't get my good name back, and I feel like well shouldn't you stop? And she's like why should I stop 'cause I can't get my name back. And I'm like, yes you can! I mean, you can stop now. You stop before you get in too deep because she's already done enough stuff. So I feel like she should stop now before she gets in too deep. And she's been like, she's like, "I'm a ho and I know it." And when I told her she was a little nasty, she was like "Well I don't care what nobody say, if I'm a ho."

EQUALIZERS1: I have like tons of friends that have had kids or are pregnant now and I mean I'm just like you know you might need to calm that down. I had a friend that just had a baby and then she was in the hospital still talking about I'm still gonna be a ho, I'm still gonna be a ho, and nobody out here telling me that I need to stop. And it's true, 'cause her mom's never home and she don't know who her daddy is, stuff like that so . . .

This animated exchange offers much to unpack. The daughters both disapproved of the boys' negative evaluation of other girls and in some cases the ability to decide the terms of the relationships. But they also had a contradictory sensibility about girls' role and participation in these gendered dynamics. They held girls just as or even more responsible than boys. They also agreed with the observations that some actions could make one a "ho," as defined by others. The anecdote that Equalizers4 shares about one of her friends is sobering. A girl is unable to "get her good name back" due to a social labeling gendered power dynamic. In discussing these challenges, it is clear the girls don't yet have compelling ways to talk back to the culture or mobilize counternarratives about girls' sexuality.

Daughters were often highly critical of the clothing that girls wore and how this contributed to boys' estimations of them. This contradictory attitude emerged strongly across the focus groups. We continue with the Equalizers. Equalizers1 offers the observation that some girls may engage in unwanted sexual activity to feel loved:

EQUALIZERS1: I don't think females should be like that toward themselves, but I feel like that's how society makes females feel.

EQUALIZERS4: A lot of boys make girls feel like it's the right thing to do, you're supposed to do it and if this is not done you're just like an outcast and you not supposed to talk and stuff like that. I mean it hits especially once you get to high school. People are just like you know, you ain't done it yet? What's wrong with you, you ain't like the rest of us. And, a lot of girls do it just to get attention.

EQUALIZERS1: Yeah, 'cause I saw some stuff yesterday that I really did not want to see, like females they—

EQUALIZERS3: —they come to school dressed like any old lady and they act however they want to.

EQUALIZERS1: I hate it, I feel like when girls are like that they make a name for everyone, like for every girl. Like I have a friend, I love her to death, we've been friends for a long time but she's just like, when it comes down to wearing certain things that you shouldn't wear and doing certain things, she does do it, like she wears little skimpy skirts—

EQUALIZERS3: —I have a friend like that too—

EQUALIZERS1: —and like, little tube tops and she's all around boys shaking her butt in front of them, like it's okay to shake your butt at a party, but like I mean, she does it in skirts, and she took this picture and she was bent over and she had on a skirt and she just doesn't . . .

EQUALIZERS4: Doesn't have respect for herself.

EQUALIZERS1: [Agrees]

[Others agree and suggest that boys take advantage of girls.]

Although they did not like the policing of girls' bodies by boys and authority figures, the way they viewed girls' own participation is often linked to behavior about dress and actions. The Moderates responded to the scenario much like the Equalizers did. They explored ideas of how girls are viewed unfairly by others and the media. In quotes that follow, as was typical of the other groups, the conversation quickly turned toward the girls' behavior.

Several people shouted that what the hypothetical boyfriend asks of his girlfriend is stupid:

MODERATES3: Nowadays, honestly, and I tell you no lie, do y'all remember that movie *Mean Girls*?

ALL: Yeah!

MODERATES3: . . . the exact same scenario, nowadays it's okay for a girl to dress like a ho on Halloween and don't nobody think nothing about it. But if she dress like that every single day she's considered a ho. Now why is it that one day, why is it that one night that you can dress like a ho and not considered to be a ho because it's a costume, but when you go out and do it on a Saturday night she considered a ho? What is with that?

MODERATES5: You want to know our response, what we would say to our friend? Are you out of your mind!? I mean, that's just, based on my friends, I would hope that none of them would even consider [others interject "Thank you!" and "For real!"] that based on, not even how they feel about themselves but how much women had to go through for [their] rights and you're going back to "Oh,

I have a pimp I need to get him his money by Friday?" I would be a little upset that you would even consider going out, not even doing it behind closed doors, but going out in public like that . . .

[Delivered with emotion]

MODERATES4: [interrupts] Exactly, because nowadays, it's like every single thing that a girl do, a girl can say, you know, ooh I kissed this boy and she's considered as a ho, but you know if you gonna dress like one knowing that there's a lot of people that talk about that term, and then dress like that and go to a party, and then come back and think that everything is good and jolly and everything, people's gonna talk about that and it's gonna hurt your feelings, so that's a bad idea.

MODERATES2: I also think, along with what she said, that dressing up like a ho is, to me, and maybe I'm the only one, I think I'm the only one who feels this way, but that's like an incident of rape waiting to happen. Because it's like, you got the dude, he the pimp. You goin' to a party full a whole bunch of people and you dressed like a ho. What guy do you know that's not gonna grab you and grope you that you know he not goin' to do that? Honestly.

MODERATES4: Wearing that outfit. [Others nod]

MODERATES2: Wearing that outfit. That's like you're basically asking somebody to come take advantage of me, because you're basically putting yourself out there . . . Me and my friends, we call each other, oh you ho, you know that kind of thing, and we joke about stuff like that. But that, to go out there and actually dress like that and actually pursue that you are, that's like saying hey, I'm here, I'm open, I have on no clothes, come get me.

MODERATES4: Yeah, and then you with your boyfriend he's dressed like a pimp and you might think that you trust him but there's gone be a room in that party and he's gonna want to take you in there and do something with you and you might not be ready for it.

MODERATES5: I mean, I'm not even gonna go that far, because that's, that's using your imagination a little bit, but him even wanting to dress like a pimp and have you as a hooker is showing you a little bit of how his mind works . . . because a pimp is someone that's over you that's telling you to do this and think less of yourself [and] to get him money and material things. So that's telling you he doesn't think of me as much as I thought.

MODERATES3: That and what do you think his friends are gonna say? I wonder what she gone do after you leave that party! Come on, how you think he gone talk to his friends about the situation?

MODERATES4: What do you think his friends will say when he is in the locker room with them?

MODERATES5: Oh, you got your girl working the corner! Da duh duh.

ALL: Yeah.

MODERATES4: It's not just his friends, it's also other people who might not even know you, and they see you dressed like that and it's like they get the thought in their mind, oh she's a ho, she's a ho, she's a ho, regardless if she dress like that or not [all the time], they still gone have that thought in their mind.

. . .

MODERATES2: Yeah, just basically think twice about what you do.

They went on to question how the girl would be able leave the house dressed a certain way and whether her mother and parents would approve. Soon after, a recent concert that several of the girls had attended was mentioned and again clothing was discussed:

MODERATES5: Y'all know MegaJam just happened, did you see what some of those girls were wearing to MegaJam?

[Majority of the girls had attended]

ALL: Yeah!

MODERATOR: What's MegaJam?

MODERATES5: It's like a big concert a lot of artists come to, a bunch of rappers [cross-talk with discussion and excitement over certain rappers] and I guess, I don't know what made them [think] like oh yeah, surely they'll pull me out of the audience if I have this on. But I would see girls wearing ridiculous outfits, like short shorts, like stuff looks like underwear to me, and I'm like you wearing that outside?

. . .

MODERATES1: Um, I don't think my friend would even go for that, but if that was my friend like I would really like wanna talk to her 'cause I'd think she had some kind of self-esteem issues being that she would let her boyfriend dress her up like a ho. Yeah, like you gotta have some kind of dignity or pride in yourself. I think there would be something wrong with that relationship.

MODERATES3: Or self-esteem period, because I know for girls now it's hard to live up to what you see on TV, so trying to even pursue that, 'cause what those girls go through to even get in them videos is crazy.

MODERATES4: Ain't no tellin' what they do.

In discussing the concert, the girls mirrored similar ideas about mothers' perceptions about girls' self-presentation through clothing. These daughters also understood that the media industry has an effect on their lives. As Moderates3 noted,

I know a lot of girls now are doing it just to do it and to feel loved because they don't feel that kind of love at home. That and what they see on TV, they think it's all great and stuff, they see it on TV because it's portrayed as like, with sex now there's like, there's a car commercial with a girl sitting on the car in a bathing suit, so basically they're putting it out there like if you get this car this is what you gone get, like that sexy girl in a bathing suit, knowing that's not what you gone get, you just gone get a whole bunch of car insurance.

The Equalizers also discussed the media's effect on what is normalized for girls' and boys' behavior:

EQUALIZERS4: The videos they really don't help, because I mean you see all the girls and their butts on TV, and boys are sitting there saying yeah that's how I want my girl to act, and so girls are just like oh he just said that so I got to go out here and dress just like she dresses. I mean my mom and dad are always telling me to be your own person and if a boy likes you for how you are now, then that's okay but when he starts trying to change you then that's when you leave him alone.

They then also talked about how much boys can influence what they and their friends might wear in school:

EQUALIZERS1: Oh, I had a boyfriend y'all he used to tell me like, uh, like one day I came to school I wasn't feeling good at all, I felt real bad. And he was like you need to go home! He was like nobody don't need to see you like that and dududu, he's just running off at the mouth about how . . . and I was like wow! Yeah.

EQUALIZERS3: That is like how they say boys think that if you don't wear a short skirt to school, if you don't wear tight pants to school, if you ain't showing everything, then they really don't need you, and they're gonna tell you hey, you ain't looking right today, you need to go home. Those boys are just honest with you, they don't care. I mean they lie sometimes but sometimes when it comes to like how you dress, boys is like your boyfriend will be there and he'll be like hey, that is the ugliest thing I've seen you in, you need to go home and change that.

They discussed this for a while and then returned to other women and girls' dress and behavior:

EQUALIZERS4: My mama always told me, a man wants to guess a little bit, about what you got on under your clothes, a man wants to guess. People look at a girl with a short skirt on and they say well she easy, she's wearing a little bitty skirt. So I feel like the way you dress really is how much a person is gonna respect you and if you're walking around looking half naked like you got on a bathing suit, a boy is not gonna respect you, he's gonna look at everything else you got except for your face.

EQUALIZERS1: Well I think a lot of girls get that mainly from the media, but a lot of women don't dress like they're supposed to, a lot of women just put everything out there. And I'm not trying to be mean or nothing, but it seems like it's a lot of ugly girls that, a lot of boys are like I don't want you or stuff like that or boys try put them down, a lot of girls that have been raped and stuff like that, they're just like you know I don't got nothing else to lose, why don't I just dress like this and maybe he'll like me and stuff like that. But that ain't the right way with boys.

In this extended set of quotes, we see the previously identified patterns emerge. Throughout most of the focus groups, girls tended to reserve their harshest judgmental criticism for other girls making comments specifically about clothing (i.e., type of clothing and body size) and not acting "lady-like" or gender-appropriate. In many cases their evaluations seemed to mirror many mothers' comments about how they perceived girls. We can see the influence of mothers' focus on similar issues and the rules of respectability politics. Interestingly, even though the Experts as a whole were not one of the groups that talked extensively about dress and behavior, their daughters embraced much of this evaluative language. This suggests that these negative ideas about girls are threaded throughout everyday culture (as many recognized), their peer groups, and family members.

The daughters acknowledged the spaces that were set for them by men and boys yet were unable to imagine different spaces for themselves. We also see a more cavalier attitude expressed by some of the daughters with regard to issues of sexual assault and harassment. In some instances, daughters employ victim-blaming language that ties girls' treatment by others to what they wear. One consequence of the internalization of these norms is that girls who are victimized and sexually assaulted may not come forward to their friends or engage in victim blaming toward sexual survivors.

Conclusion

The themes presented here amplify what has been described in other work on African American mother and daughter communication about sexuality. The majority of the research has focused on adult daughters and their recall of communication from their mothers. The themes raised here help us understand how these daughters are making sense of their mothers' messages at an earlier stage of development. It also charts girls' interest in and curiosity about their bodies and the messages about sexuality that they have to navigate.

African American mother and daughter communication around sexuality is often fraught with challenges. Many mothers in this research believe that they have broken with some of the confining norms that they experienced with their own mothers from discussing sexuality and sexual health with them. However, daughters experience some of the same challenges that their mothers faced in acquiring sexual health knowledge. This research suggests a mismatch with mothers' perceptions of easy and open communication about sexual health and sexuality with their daughters. Although many mothers saw themselves as generally more open and receptive to taking about sexual health (and health in general) compared to their mothers, daughters did not believe they could get accurate, nonjudgmental information from their mothers. More than half of girls across the groups did not feel like they could talk to their mothers. Reviewing the mothers' narratives, it is clear that mothers *are* communicating with daughters about sexuality and sexual health. When we probe further into the nature of that communication, I would argue that this communication is often experienced as unsatisfying by the daughters. This communication is often fragmented, negative, or incomplete. This research also suggests that mothers are using outdated gendered scripts that exclusively focus on daughters' virginity that do not take into account other potential high-risk sexual activities that their daughters may engage in. The mothers' messages may scare girls away from wanting to ask information about not only sex but also how their bodies are changing and developing during puberty.

We see that daughters were proactively seeking information about how to navigate sexual relationships and experiences. They sought information from a variety of sources if they felt their mothers would not be supportive of them. They may have turned to a sister, aunt, female friend, or the Internet, or any combination of these. Daughters wanted to be able to talk about a range of sexual health issues with their mothers. Daughters expressed the desire for information and skill-building around communication. For daughters who did not have other adults to turn to for information about sexual health, it was not clear where or how they will obtain helpful and accurate knowledge about sexual health, STDs, and HIV prevention information other than turning to the Internet.

An important theme was how daughters were aware of gender bias in the form of sexual double standards, both in the home with siblings and in larger culture. They grappled with how gender bias affects themselves and their peers.

The cultural and social landscape that African American girls face is one that offers few representations of what we would call sex-positive healthy role models. The politics of respectability, hypersexualization of media, and peer culture create an intense tripartite disparity. A discussion of playing pimps and hos or prostitutes and casual references was already very much in the daughters' lexicons. Mothers worried about their daughters being "contaminated" by other girls' behavior. But, in these narratives we can see that many daughters had internalized negative perceptions of other girls both in terms of behavior and dress. Girls expressed contradiction and tension as they discussed the scenario. They disliked boys' negative and controlling attitudes toward girls' dress and conduct. Despite voicing those concerns and acknowledging challenges, they also held girls to the standard set by boys and masculinist culture. They wanted the girls to understand that there are rules that they all must live by (as unfair as they might deem them to be) and violating them comes at a social cost.

In the wake of the #MeToo movement and #SayHerName, communities are being called to account for the perpetuation of violence against Black girls and women. Several of the ideas that daughters expressed about what was allowable to be done to girls is troubling and sets the stage for Black girls to be complicit in their own victimization. Overcoming victim blaming is a mighty task for American culture, and it is one that has taken center stage within the last few years with the #MeToo movement and attention to the assault of young people in high school and campus contexts. Challenging taken-for-granted norms about sexuality and sexual violence in the lives of African American girls need attention, as the continual shaming of girls around gendered expectations has negative ramifications for their self-esteem and efficacy.

6

Resolutions

Black women are saying loud and clear what they think, feel, believe and do about their health. The problem is, few in the research, medical and policy community have bothered to listen—until now.
—Linda Goler Blount, President and CEO, *Black Women's Health Imperative*

The importance and value of highlighting systemic inequities of African American women's and girls' health as a fundamental issue of public policy and part of a necessary political struggle has emerged as a salient issue in the last decade and a half. Activist scholars seek to push beyond status quo assumptions and limitations in how various disciplines have framed, ignored, or mispresented African American women's and girls' health. Consequently, they have sparked new questions across multiple domains of inquiry. The activism and theory-building by Black women and girls participating in multiple protest formations (i.e., Black Lives Matter, #SayHerName, #Black Girl Magic) have purposively articulated the consequences of living through intersectional identities and their contribution to negative health outcomes.

My work steps into this highly creative and turbulent moment offering a fruitful examination of health opportunities and challenges as *lived* through a specific community of African American mothers and daughters. I take as my starting point the assumption that mothers and daughters discuss a variety of health issues and mothers, over time, communicate ideas and values to their daughters about health. I also take as my starting point that mothers and daughters negotiate and make sense of their health in complex ways that have not been fully explored by scholars. Analysis of their experiences complicates and enriches our understanding of the lives of African American mothers and their adolescent daughters in the southern United States, specifically the role of internal and external barriers they face in pursuing a state of health and well-being. My analysis also pays particular attention to sexual health and how mothers understand and manage their daughters' transition into young womanhood.

By situating their narratives together and at times in conversation with each other, a task not commonly undertaken by scholars, we are able to see how similar some of the tensions, dilemmas, and contradictions are across both of their lives. Such a dual reference point provides a deeper and enriched perspective on the complexity of health and engages the sociological concept of linked lives. In analyzing the impact of interlocking forms of oppression on mother and daughter health, this work seeks to move from the traditional disciplinary silos of unidimensional analysis to one that is contextual and systems-based.[1]

Exploring the "worldview" of focus groups has been an analytical strategy to make sense of the data. These group interviews provide a pointed but brief picture of the lives of these mothers and daughters. Although focus groups do not lend themselves to generalizability, the themes about health that emerged from the data are not divorced from the evidence of enduring patterns, given various health indicators, we see in wider communities of African American women and girls. As noted in the introduction and in chapter 1, in many areas African American women's and girls' health status as compared to other groups remains a cause for concern. In moving the analytical lens between the dynamic mother and daughter groups, we see a resonant picture that exposes the structural and individual challenges that ripple throughout many families.

This research is a snapshot of the health realities of lower-middle-class and middle-class African American mothers. Eleven of the mothers are single parents, several of whom also had early pregnancies. In the mothers' narratives about their own mothers, we see a pattern of intensive (and often exhaustive) labor employment. Many of their mothers were also single parents, and additionally, some had experienced early pregnancies. In analyzing their narratives of health, we see patterns of inequality that have marked the late twentieth century. For example, we can observe the impact of multiple gender and racial formations that have shaped African American families and individuals. Low wage and intensive work outside the home shaped many African American women's lives in the early and late twentieth century.[2] The participants' mothers' families were often from the South and from rural communities. Rural communities have until recently had less access to health care than people living in urban environments. In recounting their mothers' health, many of the focus group mothers noted severe health challenges that, for some, cut their parents' lives short.

African American heterosexual women's ability to create a dual-income household has also been affected by the inequalities that brutally shape African American men's life outcomes, including access to education and steady and remunerative employment opportunities. The mothers in this research have been impacted by the long-term trends that affect African American men. All of these factors, though not discussed by the participants, contribute to the trajectory of the narratives they share about their health.

Avoiding Mother Blame

Writing analytically about mothers and daughters is fraught terrain for a researcher. Generally, mothers in society often face unfair and sexist criticism in the decisions regarding child-rearing and are held to a different and higher standard than fathers. In writing a book that examines the decision-making and communication styles of participants that belong to a marginalized group(s), I am aware of the multiple harmful, classist, and racist discourses that position African American mothers as less capable than others, especially white middle-class mothers who are still viewed as an unstated norm. Additionally, research that engages with marginalized communities rarely presents participants in enough context that constitutes a holistic analysis and can consequently overstress the challenges of that community.[3] Single motherhood, being a young parent, and/or being a parent of a young mother shaped some of the most intensely shared experiences across groups. In this work I have sought to be both faithful to the data that emerged and engage in critical self-reflexive analysis throughout. I have also highlighted and underscored areas of strength and resiliency for both mothers and daughters as gleaned through analysis.

These mothers' and daughters' actions cannot be evaluated simply in a static evaluative frame of good/bad or right/wrong. They embody the complexities of people making choices and decisions with the best information and tools they have at their disposal. These mothers, as should be evident, want the best for their daughters and themselves and exist within contemporary societal opportunities and constraints. My analysis throughout points to how the complex formations of gender, race, and class invisibly shape much of the mothers' and daughters' decision-making landscape. Indeed, as sociologist Shirley Hill notes, the pushback against exclusively negative evaluations of Black female single-parent households helps society value that "they are remarkably diverse in their resources, support networks, and the ability to raise children," ultimately rejecting the idea that "they are inherently dysfunctional."[4] Hill also notes that despite "this diversity," many single Black mothers suffer economic hardships, social isolation, and other detriments that can affect them and their children's well-being.

Inheritances and Legacies

African American mothers are located within racial and classed hierarchies that shape access to health care, experiences with medical providers, and their expectations about the "payoff" of a healthy diet and exercise.

The theme of "low investment in self" was salient across all groups. At home, if partnered or married, they often faced unstated gendered expectations about the amount and role of caretaking in the home. While the home for many African American women has been theorized as a place of self-making away from racialized normative expectations, they also must contend with sexism from male partners and husbands and heavy responsibility for labor in the household and child-rearing. Those who are single parents are confronted with the realities of long hours at home and office without much relief.

Mothers in the focus groups struggled with their health in particular ways. These include maintaining a healthy weight, cooking healthy meals at home, and exercising consistently. Several also managed chronic health conditions. They looked to medical providers, but also proactively sought out information to help with their health conditions. All mothers had access to some form of health care, mostly through their employers. Many mothers were not, however, happy or satisfied with their current health-care experiences. Many also inherited folk traditions of healing from their mothers that influenced their conceptualization of health, illness, and healing.

We see parallel issues in how daughters perceive and define their health experiences. The majority of daughters did not see themselves as healthy or define their mothers as healthy. They often used negative and evaluative language about their food choices and level of physical activity. Unlike their mothers, however, boredom (which was enticement for some to overeat) was more prominent in their narratives. They sought health information from a wide variety of sources. The inconsistent ways that their mothers practiced and communicated about health I argue constitute a health barrier for themselves and many of their daughters. Daughters were aware of the obstacles their mothers faced in most instances, including the realities of many working parents—extreme work hours, the lack of time and energy to cook healthy meals and the burden of child-rearing, and in some cases dealing with elder care. Another barrier to their health was their lack of trust and overall negative opinions of health-care providers.

When we examine sexuality, we see that mothers did not possess a wide sexual education, and for the most part they resented that fact. For many, their entry into sexuality was marked with deep regret and in some cases trauma. Discussions about their daughters often raised unprocessed emotions that surfaced in relation to their own sexual and relationship experiences. Mothers across all the focus groups drew on their own personal histories when communicating with their daughters. They wanted the best for their daughters, but in identifying possible threats, they re-inscribed the good girl/

bad girl dichotomy and respectability politics that was also reflected in how their daughters navigate their own sexual subjectivity.

One of the major risk factors for girls' health was under the radar for many mothers. This research was undertaken at the height of North Carolina's rise as a leader of southern states for overall rates of HIV/AIDS. Despite ongoing public service announcements about the risks of HIV/AIDS and the importance mothers placed on their daughters' STD risk, the mothers in the focus groups did not view the potential HIV risk to their daughters as a significant concern. One explanation of this can be that overriding these concerns was their focus on virginity. This might be a feature of the peer networks and church communities that several of the mothers participated in.

For African American girls at the precipice of womanhood, their lives unfolded within similar constraints as their mothers', despite many societal changes. They must contend with rigid sexual scripts that dictate what is considered appropriate behavior. They, like their mothers, operate within a context of sexism and racism that can constrain African American girls' safe pursuit of sexual autonomy and identity. As other scholars have noted, African American girls must contend with being positioned within dominant and African American culture as hypersexual.[5] Being positioned in this way contributes to their confusion and frustration in the expression of sexuality.

Daughters experienced their mothers' communication about relationships, sexuality, and intimacy in a variety of ways. Sometimes such communication was viewed as helpful and wanted, but many times daughters perceived it as intrusive, combative, and judgmental. In two groups, the Loners and Distrusters, these issues were pronounced because of already seemingly frayed relationships with mothers. Many daughters were acutely aware that their mothers had experienced challenging relationship and sexual experiences.

Daughters' narratives help us to reflect on the ways that communities have done a poor job of adequately supporting girls' sexual agency and identity. And, as we can see in this work, the current social environment is shaped in a sexist way such that pleasure, curiosity, and desire are often left out of both mother and daughter sexual communication.

The daughters all attended schools in North Carolina during the time when there was a shift from teaching abstinence-only in public schools to the implementation of a choice model. Many mentioned that they found the counselors and health professionals helpful by providing them with information that was presented in a clear, nonjudgmental way. School-based sex education, however, is not a panacea. School-based sex education has been shown to also replicate bias and invisibility, especially for LGBTQ students. Despite the limitations of school-based sex education as currently practiced, I agree with Lorena Garcia in her analysis of Latina girls' navigation of school-based sex education curricula.[6] Garcia argues that a more nuanced approach that integrates girls' experiences and moves away from a gender-based model that assumes stereotypes about masculinity and femininity could be empowering for more girls.

What emerges clearly from the focus group narratives is that daughters are agents; they are actively seeking sexual knowledge and they are turning to multiple sources. They often do not turn to their mothers. For daughters who have access to speak with helpful adults who are willing to discuss sexual health topics, they may be able to gain information that will help them make informed decisions. This was the case for several girls across the focus groups. What is unclear and concerning are how the girls in this study, who have no reliable adult figures to have discussions with will fare.

Future Directions

The nation has been stuck in a conversation about health care that has changed little over the past decade. During President Obama's time in office, the Affordable Care Act emerged as a way to cover the many millions of people without insurance and to encourage disease prevention and stream-line efficiency. The Trump years have seen a reversal and undermining of ACA. Moving forward, however, without strong and consistent measures that account for the complex ways race, class, and gender structure health access and experiences with providers will leave many African American women's and girls' needs ignored or underserved.

Moreover, COVID-19's emergence and spread, in the United States, during 2020 has made visible the long-standing patterns of structural inequalities that underscore the negative health realities that face Black girls and women. We are only at the beginning of understanding the ways that COVID-19 exploited the long-standing histories of "low-wage essential work and care-taking" activities that define the daily realities for many Black women and women of color.[7] The cumulative and structural realities that affect the African American mothers in this study, like other African American mothers nationally, are multiple and are not easily corrected without significant policy and political interventions.[8]

In traveling around the country over the years discussing this research, I often ask audience members if they remember their own conversations about health, sex, and sexuality with adults when they were adolescents. They often get a rather pained look on their face, and their body language changes. I find this interesting, as I am not a parent and had a mother who could talk about things with ease. Of course, I cannot generalize from a series of presentations to both academics and civic organizations, but it does remind me of the expectations we have of parents and communication, especially in the area of sexuality. Parents are often thought to be the best and only arbiters of imparting information and guidance about sexuality. When I started this work, I assumed that, too. Indeed, the health literature often supports this framework. My work with mothers and daughters suggests that many parents find this emotional work difficult and uncomfortable to undertake, and it often yields varying results.

Strengthening mother and daughter communication, however, especially in the area of sexuality, is an important short-term goal. This is difficult to do without recognition and support for mothers' own level of difficulty, trauma, and shame in dealing with sexual experiences. During the study period, the majority of the mothers were in their late 30s to 40s, thus a mix of Gen-Xers and Millennials. Although sexual assault was not mentioned by participants, given national statistics and the findings of the #MeToo Movement, we cannot ignore that many African American women have experienced some type of sexual trauma and much of that bodily experience still remains hidden and unexamined. The National Intimate Partner and Sexual Violence Survey "revealed that 41% of Black women experienced sexual coercion and other forms of unwanted sexual contact."[9] One possible way to support African American women (whether mothers or not) on these issues is to provide safe, positive, and supportive spaces that offer nurturance and nonjudgement, founded in the model of "sistercircles." Sistercircles are intentional spaces that are convened by Black women interested in supporting each other on vital issues.

There is enormous need for sistercircles and created sanctuary spaces for Black women to gather to support each other, especially with regard to cultivating healthy sexuality. These formations can be in the context of community organizations, support groups, and other spaces that are accessible and have community buy-in. Such spaces can be peer-led or involve trained counselors and facilitators. Mothers, in my research, desired more support from their communities to help them with guiding their daughters through young womanhood from a position of strength.

Additionally, a hard look at the ways in which Black girls are viewed within Black communities is warranted. I propose an African American mother and daughter national summit to address a vision of collective Black girlhood and wellness. This national summit would bring together various collectives and groups that have been mobilizing under several political and social formations (e.g., #SayHerName). The emphasis of the summit would focus on the well-being of Black girls, and one component would be revisiting mother and daughter relationships.

ACKNOWLEDGMENTS

This book was determined to be written in its own way and in its own time. Given that I have been a scholar for more than 20 years and have written several books, I believed that my process for writing this book would resemble what had come before. I believed that I could command words when needed and shape them as I had on so many prior occasions. The process of writing this book was *nothing* like any of my other books. As the memoirist Dani Shapiro has said in interviews, "Every book is its own mountain to climb." Climbing this book's mountain demanded new and unique levels of perseverance and emotional fortitude that I had not previously summoned. It also required a legion of helpers, supporters, and encouragers as I scaled this book's mountain. I give thanks to those people and institutional spaces here.

I am indebted to the University of North Carolina–Chapel Hill's Institute for the Arts and Humanities for the research support they provided while writing this book. Workshopping my ideas with the other Fellows played a crucial role both at the beginning of the book's conceptualization and toward its completion. My Faculty Fellowship in 2012 was revelatory as the Fellows helped me realize that I wanted to write a much bigger book involving African American mother and daughter health that not was solely focused on HIV/AIDS. Returning as a Fellow in spring 2020 after a substantial period of solitary writing, it was invigorating and useful to hear Fellows' perspectives on the introduction as the book was nearing completion. A special thanks goes to Tanya Shields, Faculty Fellow and colleague in the Department of Women's and Gender Studies, for her warmth, support, and the lending of books and resources during my final push of writing.

I am grateful to readers of early drafts of book proposals and chapters as well as conversations with Ruth Nicole Brown, Kia Caldwell, Billye Sankofa Waters, Jennifer Fish, Karen Tice, Julia Jordan Zachery, and Pat Parker.

Thanks to my academic writing group members, Karolyn Tyson and Lisa Pearce. I have benefited enormously over the decade that we have been working together from your critical insights, perceptive reading, and effective feedback.

Several colleagues at UNC–Chapel Hill made themselves available for discussions about the challenges and joys of book writing as a midcareer faculty member, including Mark Crescenzi, Todd Ochoa, David Kiel, and Mark Katz, that were illuminating. Colleagues Karen Booth and Jennifer Ho always provided encouraging words about the book's progress. Kia Caldwell and Pat Parker are not only some of the most inspiring and generous colleagues that I have ever known, they are fantastic friends. Thanks for making me laugh, asking me the tough questions, keeping our "sista lunches" going despite impossible schedules, and assuring me that this book would get written and have something to contribute. Pamela Lothspeich, colleague, friend, and former neighbor, made sure to check in with me regularly about the book's development. I am so appreciative of the many pep talks she delivered and the kindness that she showered on me during the multiple phases of drafting and revision.

I'm profoundly grateful to have worked with Academic Coaching and Writing led by Sally Jensen. Through ACW's approach, I cultivated and sustained healthy writing habits that contributed to the completion of this book. My thanks also go to Libby, Ken, Sarah, and most especially Chin-Sun, who moderated ACW's online "Writing Room." Their good cheer and brief side conversations through Zoom chat always made me look forward to showing up for the day's work.

My thanks also go to Easton's Nook, an enchanting writing retreat tucked away in Newark, New Jersey that I discovered when I needed it the most.

I am fortunate to have worked with Kim Greenwell and thankful for her editing assistance in the final stages of the book.

Over the years, I've worked with a fantastic and hardworking cadre of research assistants, and I would like to acknowledge them: Daiysa Smith, Sol Pederson, Brennan Lewis, Sloan Godbey, Emma Heasley, Faith Virago, Cosima Hernandez, Eman Chowdhury, and Tomiko Hackett.

I am indebted to coach (and now friend) Moira Killoran who tirelessly and with compassion and great skill helped me focus on what was most important to achieve daily, weekly, and monthly during the several semesters of book drafting. I can say unequivocally that this book would not exist without her. Thank you!

I am extremely grateful to the mothers and daughters who shared their perspectives in my focus groups and made themselves available to me so that I could learn from them.

I offer my deep appreciation to my editor, Ilene Kalish, who believed in this project from the beginning and never wavered. Thanks to the anonymous reviewers, whose feedback made the book stronger, and the staff at New York University Press who guided the manuscript through the production process.

Then there are dear friends who bolstered and cheered me on throughout this long journey. I want to recognize and thank Lynne Degitz for offering unwavering support and always being willing to listen to "narration" (that sometimes looked like outright complaining) about how I was doing. We do the hard things, Lynne! Thanks to Jodi Sandfort, who always helped me hold the bigger vision. Thanks to Cheryl Radeloff, Vaughn Upshaw, Kathleen Guidroz, and Jodi O'Brien for being steady, positive influences in my life.

Timothy Dane Keim, my partner of 20 years (and now fiancé) has routinely been witness to the laborious and definitely unglamorous process of writing an academic book. Several books in, I'm grateful he still showers me with such patience and good cheer. With this book, he went above and beyond the call of duty as a loyal and loving champion. Your love is something that I can bask in, count on, and am daily awed by. Thank for you everything.

APPENDIX

Methodological Notes

PROFILE OF RESEARCH PARTICIPANTS' CHARACTERISTICS

A short survey was administered to each mother before she participated in the focus groups. The survey included background questions about the mothers' educational level, income, and length of stay in North Carolina.

24 mother and daughter pairs participated in the focus groups. Out of the 24 mother-daughter pairs, five mothers lived below a $25,000 annual income level. 11 mothers were married, two were divorced, and 11 were single. Of these same mothers, the majority had graduated from high school and college and two held advanced degrees. A majority of the participants were born and raised in North Carolina.

COLLECTING AND ANALYZING THE DATA

Recruitment

This project was approved through UNC–Chapel Hill's Institutional Review Board. Women who identified as mothers and as African American in a large North Carolina city and surrounding suburbs were recruited. The designation of the category of mother was flexible and included women who were biological mothers but also those who were guardians or who had primary responsibilities for a young woman. This flexibility was informed by Patricia Hill Collins's understanding of "othermothering" that happens in many Black communities where patterns of caring relations are not limited to biological ties.[1] The daughters that were recruited were between the ages of 12 and 18. All of the participating mothers had only one daughter at the time of research that met the age criteria. The mothers were recruited for a discussion about health concerns for themselves and their daughters and to share perceptions about their daughters' entry into adolescence. Their daughters were recruited for a discussion about their health and what it means to be a young woman. My recruitment strategy included multiple postings through social networks, community centers, OB-GYN and pediatrician offices, Department of Health programs, and snowball sampling.

Focus Group Protocol

Focus groups were conducted using a series of open-ended questions and vignettes. Each mother and daughter received at $25 gift card for participation; additionally, each dyad selected a book of choice on health and wellness from selections offered. After the mothers completed the background survey, the daughters and mother went into separate rooms for sessions that lasted approximately two hours to three hours. No identifying information was used during the focus group sessions, and participants were asked to keep the discussion private.

To maintain confidentiality, I have assigned pseudonyms to study participants (when identified individually), the people they referenced, and institutions and organizations they referenced. Also, I have altered small features of physical descriptions of participants when necessary as a safeguard against possible identification.

I supplemented this work with participant observation in various settings that included African American mothers and daughters (i.e., community events) and informal interviews with several mothers and daughters who participated in the study. This component of my embeddedness allowed me to complement and clarify some of the information that was percolating up through the focus groups.

This work emerged from a collaboration that I led with key staff members in a local arts-based organization, and several graduate students from Duke University and the University of North Carolina–Chapel Hill, all of whom identified as Black women. From the beginning we thought of our work together as a community-engaged participatory project that sought to take a strengths-based approach (as opposed to a deficit model approach) in investigating the questions: What's already working well with African American mother and daughter communication in relation to health and sexuality? What are their health needs that are not being addressed? How can we support and make visible African American mothers and daughters defining their own health needs? And where might there be an opportunity for strengthening skills that could prevent (or reduce) HIV/AIDS? When I began this work in the early 2000s, the reality of the high rates of HIV/AIDS rates in North Carolina (some of the highest in the country) were front and center in my mind.

Unlike many other types of qualitative research, the researcher's self-reflexivity as a part of the analysis can vary widely in the presentation of focus group research. I have chosen to bring myself into the discussion in the introduction. From the comments that I received both before, during, and after the interviews from the mothers, the fact that I, as a Black woman, was the lead researcher on this project mattered. They told me and the team they would probably not have participated if there wasn't a Black woman in the room asking questions, nor would they have been as open and forthcoming. Although I mentioned during the recruitment calls that I was an African American woman, on the day the focus groups met, mothers reiterated their relief to see an African American–led research team. They also appreciated that we as a team had created an engaging space for them to discuss these issues. Although I shared racial and gender characteristics with the participants, especially the mothers, I didn't share the life experience of mothering. As a team we wanted to acknowledge and honor the mothering wisdom in the room, so we decided that when possible, the lead moderator for the mother focus groups would also be a mother, usually a role taken up by one of the staff members of the partnering community organization. Occupying different vantage points throughout the research process as lead researcher, moderator, and notetaker offered a richness to my analysis of the materials.

NOTES

INTRODUCTION

1 See Barlow and Dill 2018; Arriola, Borba, and Thompson 2007; Dill In Press; Blount 2018; Crenshaw 2015; Crenshaw, Ocen, and Nanda 2015.
2 See Davis 1983; Blount 2018; Barlow and Dill 2018.
3 Harding 2013.
4 Elder 1987.
5 Ibid.
6 Thornberry, Freeman-Gallant, and Lovegrove 2009.
7 Stephens and Phillips 2003; Townsend 2008.
8 Collins 1990; Hill 2005.
9 US Bureau of the Census 2016.
10 See Rainey et al. 1999; Strauss and Knight 1999; Ziol-Guest and Dunifon 2014.
11 Centers for Disease Control 2012.
12 See Inrig 2011.
13 Centers for Disease Control 2012; Southern AIDS Coalition 2012.
14 Berger 2004; Hader et al. 2001; Quinn 1993.
15 Caldwell and Matthews 2015; Watkins-Hayes 2011.
16 See Stephens and Phillips 2003; Arnowitz, Rennells, and Todd 2005; Townsend 2008; Dennis and Wood 2012.
17 Crenshaw et al. 2015
18 Kumanyika 2018b.
19 Ogden et al. 2012.
20 Centers for Disease Control 2012.
21 Hill 2005; Schultz and Mullings 2005; Weber 2005.
22 Weber 2005; Mullings and Schultz 2005.
23 See Davis 1983; Avery 1989; White 1994.
24 See Davis 1983.
25 Collins 1990, 2004.
26 See Christian 1985; Spillers 1984.
27 See Collins 1990, 2004; Bennett and Dickerson 2001; Hobson 2005. Also see Bailey 2016.
28 Hobson 2005: 14.
29 Ibid.
30 See Jewell 1993; Berger 2004; Hobson 2005. Also see Hancock 2004; Jordan-Zachery 2008; Collins 1990; Simms 2001.
31 Collins 2000: 101.
32 Barlow and Dill 2018; Blount 2018.
33 Barlow and Dill, 2018: 221.
34 See also Blount 2018; Kumayika 2018a.

35 See Arriola et al. 2007.

36 Price 2007; Lau 2011. Also see Chadiha and Brazelton 2012.

37 Hill 2005, 2007; Battle and Barnes 2010; Hunter, Guerrero, and Cohen 2010.

38 Brown 2012.

39 See Rose 2004.

40 See Schulz and Mullings 2005; Weber 2005.

41 Firth 2012; Kulbaga and Spencer 2017.

42 Firth 2012.

43 Obama 2012.

44 Ibid.

45 Firth 2012.

46 Kulbaga and Spencer 2017.

47 The only other African American woman who occupied such a public role in America's health is Faye Wattleton, president of Planned Parenthood from 1978 to 1992. She transformed the organization and was often on the front lines on debates about abortion, birth control, and women's health.

48 Collins 1990; Hill 2008.

49 Obama 2013.

50 Kulbaga and Spencer 2017; Firth 2012.

51 See Popkin and Doak 1998; Young and Nestle 2002.

52 See Gard and Wright 2005; Wright and Harwood 2012.

53 Obama 2010.

54 Obama 2013.

55 Ibid.

56 Obama 2009.

57 White 2009.

58 See Lee 2009.

59 Mask 2012.

60 Thompson 1992.

61 Albers 2009.

62 Burton 2017: 65.

63 Ibid.

64 Bastién 2016.

65 See Burton 2017.

66 Evans 2017: 110.

67 Epstein, Blake, and González 2019.

68 Police were called to investigate alleged fighting at a pool party in a suburban neighborhood of McKinney, Texas. Police officer Eric Casebolt was video-recorded forcefully and violently restraining Dajerria Becton, a 15-year-old African American girl, wearing a swimsuit, on the ground. This was after Dajerria and the other group of multi-racial teens (who were invited by a resident, a young white girl) were leaving after being racially harassed by some of the other white women residents in attendance. The brutal incident was recorded by another teenage attendee. The video was released shortly after the incident and went viral. The incident sparked outrage and a public discussion of the treatment of teenagers of color (especially African Americans) by police officers. It also sparked increased awareness of the criminalization and brutalization of Black women and girls (Ritchie 2018; Macais 2018).

Becton settled with Casebolt and the city of McKinney in a federal lawsuit in May 2018. She was awarded $148,850.

69 Crenshaw et al. 2015: 7.

70 Crenshaw 2015.

71 Jackson 2014.

72 See Velazquez 2016.

73 Zachery and Harris 2019.

74 The designation of the category of mother was flexible and included women who were biological mothers but also those who were guardians or who had primary responsibilities for a young woman. This flexibility was informed by Patricia Hill Collins's (1990) understanding of "othermothering" that happens in many Black communities where patterns of caring relations are not limited to biological ties.

75 Krueger 1998: 20, 150; Harding 2013.

76 See Wilkinson 1998; Pini 2002; Ritchie and Barker 2005; Jowett and Gill 2006.

77 See Ritchie and Barker 2005; Pini 2002; Jowett and O'Toole 2006.

78 Duggleby 2005; Ritchie and Barker 2005.

79 2005: 9.

80 See Harding 2013: 160–167; Hennink 2014.

81 A best practice suggested by Harding 2013.

82 Harding 2013.

83 See Collins 1990; Berger and Guidroz 2010; Choo and Ferree 2010.

84 Choo and Ferree 2010.

85 See Choo and Ferree 2010.

CHAPTER 1. MOTHER AND DAUGHTER NARRATIVES ABOUT HEALTH, SEXUALITY, AND YOUNG WOMANHOOD

1 Maddock 2018.

2 Center for Women's Health Research 2014.

3 Maddock 2018.

4 This is a fictitious college.

CHAPTER 2. MOTHERS' HEALTH NARRATIVES

1 I am indebted to Kim Greenwell for raising this point with me.

2 Chapman, Kaatz, and Carnes 2013; DiMatteo et al. 2009.

CHAPTER 3. "I'M IN BETWEEN"

1 In political science, see Harris-Perry 2011; in public health, Woods-Giscomb 2018; sociology, Beauboeuf-Lafontant 2009.

2 While public health and the medical community are actively trying to understand the impact of race, gender, and other disparities, it has been focused on adults. More research needs to be conducted on African American girls' and young women's experiences with a variety of providers from childhood through college age. One exception is Jernigan (2019) and her focus group work with African American girls and their perceptions of medical providers' information about weight and nutrition.

CHAPTER 4. "I WANT THAT FIRST KISS TO BE PERFECT"

1 Dennis and Wood 2012.
2 Dennis and Wood 2012; Townsend 2008; Rose 2004; Stephens and Philips 2003.
3 I grew up hearing this term used, too, in reference to female sexuality. After doing some digging on Wikipedia about the origins of the term, it refers to a garment with "each of the flaps formed by the lower back of a coat, especially a tailcoat." This strikes me as ironic, given that historically it has been men who typically have worn tailcoats.
4 On Black women, see Higginbotham 1993; on inconsistent cultural messages and sexual behavior, see Karaian 2014.
5 Although two girls, out of the entire 24 daughter participants, identified as lesbian and bisexual, mothers as a whole were focused on heterosexuality.
6 Morgan 2015.

CHAPTER 5. "MOM, CAN WE TALK ABOUT SEX?"

1 In reviewing my notes across the focus groups, I don't believe that when two of the daughters said they thought sex could be labeled "traumatic" that they were specifically speaking about sexual violence that they had experienced. I believe their definition speaks more to the emotional ramifications of becoming sexually active. However, given that first sexual experiences for many girls is not always consensual, I also want to hold the possibility that this framing of sex as traumatic may grow out of conversations with their peers that could indicate sexual assault and violence. Although we did not ask girls to disclose if they were sexually active, it is also possible that these two participants could have experienced sexual assault.
2 My sense, gleaned from informal interviews with girls (not officially part of the study), was that deviance from heterosexual behavior was discouraged and sometimes even punished by parents, especially mothers.
3 Gibson 2007.
4 The scenario was crafted by the research team based on a real-life incident that had occurred with one of the team members in her interaction with a young woman.

CHAPTER 6. RESOLUTIONS

1 Kumanyika 2018a.
2 Hill 2008, 2005.
3 Okafor 2018.
4 Hill 2005: 204.
5 Stephens and Phillips 2003.
6 Garcia 2013.
7 Lindsey 2020.
8 See Hill 2005.
9 West and Johnson 2013.

APPENDIX

1 Collins 1990.

BIBLIOGRAPHY

Albers, Susan. 2009. "Precious, Sexual Abuse & Eating Disorders." *Psychology Today.* December 28. www.psychologytoday.com.

Aronowitz, Teri, Rachel E. Rennells, and Erin Todd. 2005. "Heterosocial Behaviors in Early Adolescent African American Girls: The Role of Mother-Daughter Relationships." *Journal of Family Nursing* 11(2): 122–139.

Arriola, Kimberly R. Jacob, Christina P. C. Borba, and Winifred Wilkins Thompson. 2007. "The Health Status of Black Women: Breaking Through the Glass Ceiling." *Black Women, Gender + Families* 1, no. 2 (Fall): 1–23.

Avery, Byllye. 1989. "Black Women's Health: A Conspiracy of Silence." *Sojourner* 14(5): 15.

Bailey, Moya. 2016. "Misogynoir in Medical Media: On Caster Semenya and R. Kelly." *Catalyst: Feminism, Theory, Technoscience* 2(2): 1–31.

Barlow, Jameta Nicole and LeConté J. Dill. 2018. "Speaking for Ourselves: Reclaiming, Redesigning, and Reimagining Research on Black Women's Health." *Meridians: feminism, race, transnationalism* 16(2): 219–229.

Bastién, Angelica Jade. 2016. "Why Alfre Woodard's Mariah Is *Luke Cage*'s Secret Weapon." *Vulture.* October 18. www.vulture.com.

Battle, Juan and Sandra L. Barnes, eds. 2010. *Black Sexualities: Probing Powers, Passions, Practices, and Policies.* New Brunswick, NJ: Rutgers University Press.

Beauboeuf-Lafontant, Tamara. 2009. *Behind the Mask of the Strong Black Woman: Voice and the Embodiment of a Costly Performance.* Philadelphia: Temple University Press.

Bell-Scott, Patricia, Beverly Guy-Sheftall, Jacqueline Jones Royster, Janet Sims-Wood, Miriam DeCosta-Willis, and Lucie Fultz, eds. 1993. *Double Stitch: Black Women Write about Mothers and Daughters.* New York: Perennial.

Bennett, Michael and Vanessa D. Dickerson. 2001. *Recovering the Black Female Body: Self-Representations by African American Women.* New Brunswick, NJ: Rutgers University Press.

Berger, Michele. 2004. *Workable Sisterhood: The Political Journey of Stigmatized Women with HIV/AIDS.* Princeton, NJ: Princeton University Press.

Berger, Michele and Kathleen Guidroz, eds. 2010. *The Intersectional Approach: Transforming the Academy through Race, Class and Gender.* Chapel Hill: University of North Carolina Press.

Black Women's Blueprint. 2016. "When Truth Is Justice and Not Enough: Executive Summary to the Black Women's Truth and Reconciliation Commission Report." www.blackwomensblueprint.org.

Bloor, Michael, Jane Frankland, Michelle Thomas, and Kate Robson. 2001. *Focus Groups in Social Research*. Thousand Oaks, CA: Sage Press.

Blount, Linda Goler. 2018. "The Secret to Black Women's Health: Ask, Listen, Do." *Meridians: feminism, race, transnationalism* 16, no. 2: 253–259.

Brooks, Kevin L. 2014. "Improving the Lives of Black Girls Is as Important as Saving Black Boys." *AAASCEC* (blog). September 10. https://u.osu.edu/aaascec.

Brown, Ruth Nicole. 2012. *Black Girlhood Celebration: Toward a Hip-Hop Feminist Pedagogy*. New York: Peter Lang.

Burton, Nsenga K. 2017. "Representations of Black Women's Mental Illness in the HTGAWM and Being Mary Jane." In *Black Women's Mental Health: Balancing Strength and Vulnerability*, edited by Stephanie Y. Evans, Kanika Bell, and Nsenga K. Burton, 57–74. Albany: State University of New York Press.

Caldwell, Kia and Allison Matthews. 2015. "The Role of Relationship Type, Risk Perception, and Condom Use in Middle Socioeconomic Status Black Women's HIV-prevention Strategies." *Journal of Black Sexuality and Relationships* 2(2): 91–120.

Center for Women's Health Research. 2014. "Report Card." University of North Carolina, School of Medicine. www.med.unc.edu.

Centers for Disease Control and Prevention. 2012. *Estimated HIV Incidence in the United States, 2007–2010. HIV/AIDS Surveillance Supplemental Report* 17(4): 14: 1–26.

Chadiha, Leitha A. and Jewell F. Brazelton. 2012. "Aging, Physical Health and Work and Family Role Changes among African American Women: Strategies for Conducting Life-Course Research with African American Women." In *Researching Black Communities: A Methodological Guide*, edited by James S. Jackson, Cleopatra Howard Caldwell, and Sherrill L. Sellers, 79–93. Ann Arbor: University of Michigan Press.

Chapman, Elizabeth N., Anna Kaatz, and Molly Carnes. 2013. "Physicians and Implicit Bias: How Doctors May Unwittingly Perpetuate Health Care Disparities." *Journal of Internal Medicine* 28(11): 1504–1510.

Choo, Hae Yeon and Myra Marx Ferree. 2010. "Practicing Intersectionality in Sociological Research: A Critical Analysis of Inclusions, Interactions, and Institutions in the Study of Inequalities." *Sociological Theory* 28(2): 129–149.

Christian, Barbara. 1985. *Black Feminist Criticism: Perspectives on Black Women Writers*. New York: Pergamon Press.

Collins, Patricia Hill. 2004. *Black Sexual Politics*. New York: Routledge.

———. 2000. "Gender, Black Feminism, and Black Political Economy." *ANNALS of the American Academy of Political and Social Science* 568, no. 1: 41–53.

———. 1990. *Black Feminist Thought: Knowledge, Consciousness and the Politics of Empowerment*. Boston: Unwin Hyman.

Crenshaw, Kimberlé. 2015. "Black Girls Matter." *Ms.*, Spring, 25–29.

Crenshaw, Kimberlé, Priscilla Ocen, and Jyoti Nanda. 2015. "Black Girls Matter: Pushed Out, Overpoliced and Underprotected." Center for Intersectionality and Social Policy Studies and African American Policy Forum, 1–44.

Davis, Angela. 1983. *Women, Race, and Class*. New York: Random House.

Dennis, Alexis C. and Julia T. Wood. 2012. "We're Not Going to Have This Conversation, But You Get It: Black Mother-Daughter Communication about Sexual Relations." *Women's Studies in Communication* 35(2): 204–223.

Dill, LeConté. In Press. "#CrunkPublicHealth: Decolonial Feminist Praxes of Cultivating Liberatory and Transdisciplinary Learning, Research, and Action Spaces." In *Unsettling Colonial Curriculum: Womanist and Anti-Colonial Theories and Pedagogical Interventions*, edited by Jillian Ford and Nathalia Jarmarillo. Champaign: University of Illinois Press.

DiMatteo, Robin M., Summer L. Williams, and Carolyn B. Murray. 2009. "Gender Disparities in Physician-Patient Communication Among African American Patients in Primary Care." *Journal of Black Psychology* 35(2): 204–227.

Duggleby, Wendy. 2005. "What About Focus Group Interaction Data?" *Qualitative Health Research* 15(6): 832–840.

Elder, Glen H. 1987. "Families and Lives: Some Developments in Life-Course Studies." *Journal of Family History* 12(1–3):179–199.

Epstein, Rebecca, Jamilia J. Blake, and Thalia González. 2019. "Girlhood Interrupted: The Erasure of Black Girls' Childhood." Center on Poverty and Inequality, Georgetown Law.

Evans, Stephanie. 2017. "From Worthless to Wellness: Self-Worth, Power, and Creative Survival in Memoirs of Sexual Assault." In *Black Women's Mental Health: Balancing Strength and Vulnerability*, edited by Stephanie Y. Evans, Kanika Bell, and Nsenga K. Burton, 57–74. Albany: State University of New York Press.

Evans, Stephanie Y., Kanika Bell, and Nsenga K. Burton, eds. 2017. *Black Women's Mental Health: Balancing Strength and Vulnerability*. Albany: State University of New York Press.

Firth, Jeanne. 2012. "Healthy Choices and Heavy Burdens: Race, Citizenship and Gender in the 'Obesity Epidemic.'" *Journal of International Women's Studies* 13(2): 33–50.

Garcia, Lorena. 2013. *Respect Yourself, Protect Yourself: Latina Girls and Sexual Identity*. New York: New York University Press.

Gard, Michael and Jan Wright. 2005. *The Obesity Epidemic: Science, Morality and Ideology*. New York: Routledge Press.

Gentry, Quinn M. 2007. *Black Women's Risk for HIV: Rough Living*. New York: Haworth Press.

Gibson, Faith. 2007. "Conducting Focus Groups with Children and Young People: Strategies for Success." *Journal of Research in Nursing* 12(5): 473–483.

Gilbert, Dorie J. and Ednita M. Wright, eds. 2003. *African American Women and HIV: Critical Responses*. New York: Praeger.

Hader, Shannon L., Dawn K. Smith, Janet S. Moore, and Scott D. Holmberg. 2001. "HIV Infection in Women in the United States: Status at the Millennium." *JAMA* 285(9): 1186–1192.

Hancock, Ange-Marie. 2004. *The Politics of Disgust: The Public Identity of the Welfare Queen*. New York: New York University Press.

Harding, Jamie. 2013. *Qualitative Data Analysis from Start to Finish*. Thousand Oaks, CA: Sage.

Harris-Perry, Melissa V. 2011. *Sister Citizen: Shame, Stereotype, and Black Women in America*. New Haven, CT: Yale University Press.

Hennink, Monique A. 2014. *Focus Group Discussions: Understanding Qualitative Research*. London: Oxford University Press.

Higginbotham, Evelyn Brooks. 1993. *Righteous Discontent: The Women's Movement in the Black Baptist Church, 1880–1920*. Cambridge, MA: Harvard University Press.

Hill, Shirley. 2009. "Cultural Images and the Health of African American Women." *Gender and Society* 23(6): 733–746.

———. 2008. "African American Mothers: Victimized, Vilified, and Valorized." In *Feminist Mothering*, edited by Andrea O'Reilly, 107–123. Albany: State University of New York Press.

———. 2007. "Black Families: Beyond Revisionist Scholarship." In *Shifting the Center: Understanding Contemporary Families*, edited by Susan J. Ferguson, 80–98. New York: McGraw-Hill.

———. 2005. *Black Intimacies: A Gender Perspective on Families and Relationship*. Walnut Creek, CA: AltaMira Press.

Hobson, Janell. 2005. *Venus in the Dark: Blackness and Beauty in Popular Culture*. New York: Routledge.

How to Get Away with Murder. 2014–2020. Television Show. Shona Rhimes, Producer.

Hunter, Marcus Anthony, Marissa Guerrero, and Cathy J. Cohen. 2010. "Black Youth Sexuality: Established Paradigms and New Approaches." In *Black Sexualities: Probing Powers, Passions, Practices, and Policies*, edited by Juan Battle and Sandra Barnes, 377–400. New Brunswick, NJ: Rutgers University Press.

Inrig, Stephen. 2011. *North Carolina and the Problem of AIDS: Advocacy, Politics, & Race in the South*. Chapel Hill: University of North Carolina Press.

Jackson, Chelsea A. 2014. "Developing Critical Inner Literacy: Reading the Body, the Word, and the World." PhD diss., Emory University.

Jernigan, Maryam M. 2019. "'Why Doesn't Anyone Help Us?': Therapeutic Implications of Black Girls' Perceptions of Health." *Women & Therapy* 42(3–4): 343–365.

Jewell, K. Sue. 1993. *From Mammy to Miss America and Beyond: Cultural Images and the Shaping of US Social Policy*. New York: Routledge.

Jordan-Zachery, Julia. 2008. *Black Women, Cultural Images and Social Policy*. New York: Routledge.

Jowett, Madeline and Gill O'Toole. 2006. "Focusing Researchers' Minds: Contrasting Experiences of Using Focus Groups in Feminist Qualitative Research." *Qualitative Research* 6 (November): 453–472.

Karaian, Lara. 2014. "Policing 'Sexting': Responsibilization, Respectability and Sexual Subjectivity in Child Protection/Crime Prevention Responses to Teenagers' Digital Sexual Expression." *Theoretical Criminology* 18(3): 282–299.

Krueger, Richard A. 1998. *Analysing and Reporting Focus Group Results*. London: Sage.

Kulbaga, Theresa A. and Leland G. Spencer. 2017. "Fitness and the Feminist First Lady: Gender, Race, and Body in Michelle Obama's Let's Move! Campaign." *Women and Language* 40(1): 36–50.

Kumanyika, Shiriki. 2018a. "Moving from Silos to Systems in Black Women's Health Research." *Meridians* 16: 238–258.

Kumanyika, Shiriki K. 2018b. "Supplement Overview: What the Healthy Communities Study Is Telling Us About Childhood Obesity Prevention in U.S. Communities." *Pediatric Obesity* 13(1): 3–6.

Lau, Kimberly. 2011. *Body Language: Sisters in Shape, Black Women's Fitness and Identity Politics*. Philadelphia: Temple University Press.

Lee, Felicia. 2009. "To Blacks, Precious Is 'Demeaned' or 'Angelic.'" *New York Times*, November 20.

Lindsey, Treva. 2020. "Why COVID-19 is hitting Black Women So Hard." *Women's Media Center*, April 17.

Luke Cage. 2016–2018. Television Show. Aida Mashaka Croal, Akela Cooper, and Gail Barringer. Producers.

Macais, Kelly. 2018. "Waffle House Arrest Reinforces the Pattern of Police Violence and Sexual Abuse Toward Black Women." *DailyKos*, April 27.

Maddock, Jay. 2018. "5 Charts Show Why the South Is the Least Healthy Region in the US." http://theconversation.com.

Mask, Mia. 2012. "The Precarious Politics of Precious: A Close Reading of a Cinematic Text." *Black Camera* 4(1): 96–116.

Morgan, Joan. 2015. "Why We Get Off: Moving Towards a Black Feminist Politics of Pleasure." *The Black Scholar* 45 (October): 36–46. https://doi.org/10.1080/00064246.2015.1080915.

Mullings, Leith. 1997. *On Our Own Terms: Race, Class, and Gender in the Lives of African-American Women*. New York: Routledge.

Mullings, Leith and Amy Schultz. 2005. "Intersectionality and Health: An Introduction." In *Gender, Race, Class & Health: Intersectional Approaches*, edited by Amy Schultz and Leith Mullings, 3–17. San Francisco: Jossey-Bass.

Mullings, Leith and Alaka Wali. 2001. *Stress and Resilience: The Social Context of Reproduction in Central Harlem*. New York: Springer Science & Business Media.

North Carolina Women's Health Report Card. 2009–2012. The Center for Women's Health Research. www.med.unc.edu.

Obama, Michelle. 2013. "Fireside Chat with Kelly Ripa." Interview by Kelly Ripa. March 4. Video, 34:19. www.youtube.com.

———. 2012. "Eating Healthy Isn't About How You Look." Interview. *iVillage*, August 25. Video, 3:52. www.youtube.com.

———. 2010. "Michelle Obama Combats Childhood Obesity." Interview. *Good Morning America*, February 9. Video, 6:19. www.goodmorningamerica.com.

———. 2009. "Michelle Obama on Healthy Living." Interview. *Good Morning America*, June 23. Video, 3:18. www.youtube.com.

Ogden, Cynthia L., Margaret D. Carroll, Brian K. Kit, and Katherine M. Flegal. 2012. "Prevalence of Obesity and Trends in Body Mass Index among US Children and Adolescents, 1999–2010." *JAMA* 307 (5): 483–490.

Okafor, Chinyere. 2018. "Black Feminism Embodiment: A Theoretical Geography of Home, Healing and Activism." *Meridians* 16 (2): 373–381.

Pini, Barbara. 2002. "Focus Groups, Feminist Research and Farm Women: Opportunities for Empowerment in Rural Social Research." *Journal of Rural Studies* 18: 339–351.

Popkin, Barry and Colleen Doak. 1998. "The Obesity Epidemic Is a Worldwide Phenomenon." *Nutrition Reviews* 56(4): 106–114.

Price, Kimala. 2007. "Hip Hop Feminists at the Political Crossroads: Organizing for Reproductive Justice and Beyond." In *Home Girls Make Some Noise: A Hip Hop Feminist Anthology*, edited by Gwendolyn Pough et al. Corona, CA: Parker.

Quinn, Sandra Crouse. 1993. "AIDS and the African American Woman: The Triple Burden of Race, Class, and Gender." *Health Education Quarterly* 20(3): 305–320.

Rainey, Cheryl, Richard Poling, Carol Rheaume, and Susan Kirby. 1999. "Views of Low-Income, African American Mothers about Child Health." *Family & Community Health* 22(1): 1–15.

Ritchie, Andrea. 2018. "Dajerria Becton Survived a Violent Arrest at a Pool Party and Went Viral." www.teenvogue.com.

Ritchie, Ani and Meg Barker. 2005. "Explorations in Feminist Participant-led Research: Conducting Focus Group Discussions with Polyamorous Women." *Psychology of Women Review* 7: 47–57.

Rose, Tricia. 2004. *Longing to Tell: Black Women Talk about Sexuality and Intimacy.* New York: Picador Press.

Schulz, Amy and Leith Mullings. 2005. *Gender, Race, Class & Health: Intersectional Approaches.* San Francisco: Jossey Bass.

Scott, C., D. Arthur, M. Panizo, and Roger Owen. 1989. "Menarche: The Black American Experience." *Journal of Adolescent Health Care* 10(5): 363–368.

Simms, Rupe. 2001. "Controlling Images and the Gender Construction of Enslaved African Women." *Gender & Society* 15(6): 879–897.

Southern AIDS Coalition. 2012. *Southern States Manifesto Update 2012: Policy and Recommendations.* Birmingham, AL: Southern AIDS Coalition.

Spillers, Hortense.1984. "Interstices: A Small Drama of Words." In *Pleasure and Danger*, edited by Carole Vance, 73–100. Boston: Routledge and Kegan Paul.

Stephens, Dionne P. and Layli Phillips. 2003. "Freaks, Gold Diggers, Divas and Dykes: The Socio-Historical Development of Adolescent African American Women's Sexual Scripts." *Sexuality and Culture* 7(1): 1–48.

Strauss, Richard and Judith Knight. 1999. "Influence of the Home Environment on the Development of Obesity in Children." *Pediatrics* 103(6): 1–8.

Thompson, Becky. 1992. "'A Way Outa No Way': Eating Problems among African-American, Latina, and White Women." *Gender and Society* 6(4): 546–561.

Thornberry, Terence P., Adrienne Freeman-Gallant, and Peter J. Lovegrove. 2009. "The Impact of Parental Stressors on the Intergenerational Transmission of Antisocial Behavior." *Journal of Youth Adolescence* 38(3): 312–322.

Townsend, Tiffany. 2008. "Protecting Our Daughters: Intersection of Race, Class and Gender in African American Mothers' Socialization of Their Daughter's Hetero-sexuality." *Sex Roles* 59(5–6): 429–442.

Tuck, Eve. 2009. "Suspending Damage: A Letter to Communities." *Harvard Educational Review* 79, no. 3 (Fall): 409–428.

Uhler, Tom. 2018. "Settlement Reached in Viral Video Case of McKinney Police Breaking Up a Pool Party." *Fort-Worth Star-Telegram*, May 29. www.star-telegram.com.

US Bureau of the Census. 2016. "America's Families and Living Arrangements 2016." www.census.gov.

Velazquez, Maria. 2016. "Reblog If You Feel Me: Love, Blackness, and Digital Wellness." *Yoga, The Body, and Embodied Social Change: An Intersectional Feminist Analysis*, edited by Beth Berila, Melanie Klein, and Chelsea Jackson Roberts, 175–192. Lanham, MD: Lexington Books.

Watkins-Hayes, Celeste. 2011. "Race, Respect, and Red Tape: Inside the Black Box of Racially Representative Bureaucracies." *Journal of Public Administration Research and Theory* 21(2): 233–251.

———. 2008. "The Social and Economic Context of Black Women Living with HIV/AIDS in the US: Implications for Research." In *Sex, Power, and Taboo: Gender and HIV in the Caribbean and Beyond*, edited by Rhoda Reddock et al., 33–66. Kingston, Jamaica: Ian Randle.

Weber, Lynn. 2005. "Reconstructing the Landscape of Health Disparities Research: Promoting Dialogue and Collaboration Between Feminist Intersectional and Biomedical Paradigms." In *Gender, Race, Class & Health: Intersectional Approaches*, edited by Amy Schultz and Leith Mullings, 21–59. San Francisco: Jossey-Bass.

West, Carolyn M. and Kalimah Johnson. 2013. "Sexual Violence in the Lives of African American Women." National Online Resource Center on Violence Against Women. https://vawnet.org.

White, Armond. 2009. "Review of *Precious*." *New York Press*. November 4.

White, Evelyn. 1994. 2nd ed. *The Black Women's Health Book: Speaking for Ourselves*. Boston: Seal Press.

Wikipedia. 2015. "2015 Texas Pool Party Incident." Last modified February 15, 2020. https://en.wikipedia.org.

Wilkinson, Sue. 1998. "Focus Groups in Feminist Research: Power, Interaction, and the Co-construction of Meaning." *Women's Studies International Forum* 21(1): 111–125.

Woods-Giscombe, Cheryl L. 2018. "Reflections on the Development of the Superwoman Schema Conceptual Framework: An Intersectional Approach Guided by African American Womanist Perspectives." *Meridians: Feminism, Race, Transnationalism* 16: 333–342.

Wright, Jan and V. Harwood, eds. 2012. *Biopolitics and 'The Obesity Epidemic': Governing Bodies*. New York: Routledge.

Young, L. R. and M. Nestle. 2002. "The Contribution of Expanding Portion Sizes to the US Obesity Epidemic." *American Journal of Public Health* 92(2): 246–249.

Zachery, Jordan Julia and Duchess Harris. 2019. *Black Girl Magic Beyond the Hashtag: Twenty-First Century Acts of Self-Definition*. Phoenix: University of Arizona Press.

Ziol-Guest, Kathleen M. and Rachael E. Dunifon. 2014. "Complex Living Arrangements and Child Health: Examining Family Structure Linkages with Children's Health Outcomes." *Family Relations* 63(3): 424–437.

INDEX

ABOUT THE AUTHOR

MICHELE TRACY BERGER is Associate Professor in the Department of Women's and Gender Studies at the University of North Carolina–Chapel Hill. She holds an adjunct appointment in the Department of City and Regional Planning.

Her research, teaching, and practice all focus on intersectional approaches to studying areas of inequality, especially racial and gender health disparities. This work spans the fields of public health, sociology, and women's and gender studies.

Her books include *Workable Sisterhood: The Political Journey of Stigmatized Women with HIV/AIDS*, the co-edited collections of *Gaining Access: A Practical and Theoretical Guide for Qualitative Researchers*; *The Intersectional Approach: Transforming the Academy Through Race, Class and Gender*; and the co-authored *Transforming Scholarship: Why Women's and Gender Studies Students Are Changing Themselves and the World*.

Since 2014, she has been co-investigator on a project evaluating yoga interventions in public schools and assessing their impact on adolescents, especially girls of color.